What Are Yer? Bleeder!

– DEREK HAUGHTON –

An environmentally friendly book printed and bound in England by
www.printondemand-worldwide.com

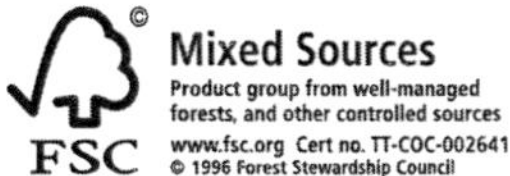

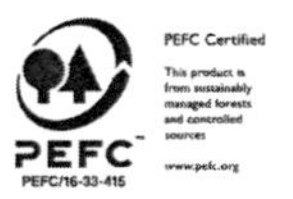

This book is made entirely of chain-of-custody materials

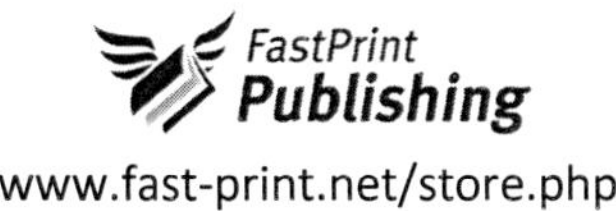

www.fast-print.net/store.php

What Are Yer? Bleeder!

All characters are fictional.
Any similarity to any actual person is purely coincidental.

ISBN 978-178035-319-7

First published 2012 by
FASTPRINT PUBLISHING
Peterborough, England.

Chapter 1

There has never been, or can ever be, a standard childhood; mine was as unique as yours, the challenges, pleasures, pains and joys as plentiful with one extra little difficulty thrown in.

I was born with severe haemophilia B owing to a damaged gene on the X-chromosome, so I can proudly boast my mutancy, sticking out my tongue at all you ordinary mortals. Don't call other haemophiliacs mutant, they won't like it.

Haemophilia was diagnosed at eighteen months old by the superb paediatrician, Mr Harry Parry-Williams, previously the stereotypical, old style surgeon Mr Bizzaro had, on my first knee bleed, decided to 'nick' the knee to see which 'fluid' was causing the swelling and pain. Doctor Vaughn, the family's G. P., had referred me to orthopaedic surgeon Bizzaro (eventually re-christened, by mum, Old Egghead) when swelling, redness, pain and fixed flexion could not be explained. Mum came to my rescue telling Bizzaro, who didn't know what to make of my problem knee and proposed the 'nicking' as a solution to his ignorance, 'No' refusing his kind offer and telling him: You're not cutting until you know what the problem is. How astute of her, it's almost as if she knew about the haemophilia! Piqued and frustrated in his mission to wield the knife Old Egghead referred me to Harry Parry-Williams, my saviour on many occasions and one of the finest practitioners and men it has been my privilege to know. The fact that I was Bizzaro's patient first gave me problems throughout my childhood as for any purely orthopaedic problem protocol demanded my being referred back to him.

I popped out into life just before the end, in Europe, of world war two and spent one night in an air-raid shelter in my uncle's garden, being carried across the road on a pillow; naturally I have no memory of this but do remember clearly the remains of two houses destroyed by bombing only three doors along the block from ours and their subsequent re-building, also two bomb-craters behind the houses, on the field known as The Dump, not a rubbish dump but where the local council chose to deposit the rubble from bombed out buildings.

The city centre had been flattened and from my push-chair I noticed the gaps between the remaining buildings and a cellar converted to static water-tank, though this is with hindsight as the image retained is only of a white tiled, perfectly rectangular hole between buildings, holding a few feet of water. A sour smell of charred timber and toasted cheese left too long under the grill gradually faded with each visit. We travelled to the city centre regularly to pay the rent and to collect a metal container of ice-cream, which would sit on the foot-rest with my legs on each side, delivering it to a local shop, why we did this I have no-one left alive to ask is able to explain. The rent office had brown floor-covering, a wooden counter and an intoxicating smell of polish which helped to cleanse the olfactory of the city centre pong.

Other early memories: Tiny dust-devils on the garden path; sparrows perching and chirping on the garden fence; wash day with a line full of billowing clothes, the larger items flapping and cracking in the wind and a wet floor where the old copper boiler had bubbled to overflow; a burned finger from reaching up on tiptoe, despite several warnings, to where mother was ironing the clothes; climbing up a sloping scaffolding plank at the re-building of the two bombed-out houses; digging into one of the borders and carrying daffodil bulbs indoors and proudly presenting them, to Mum's dismay, as onions; placing sticks in a star-shape on the path to simulate a campfire and Mum running along on The Dump trying to get a kite to fly and warning me not to run with her as I might fall, only, to my immense delight, to take a tumble herself as the words left her mouth, she wasn't hurt or resentful of my laughter at her demonstration of the truth of her words as I know I would have been.

These very early memories are without any real context or continuity but remain very vivid, as do recollections of hospitals and clinics.

For a reason that baffled me and Parry-Williams, Bizzaro once experimented by drawing venous blood from Mum and injecting it into my buttock, causing a great deal of bruising, I don't remember the struggle and the pain but Mum told me it took four nurses to hold me down! Whatever the man was up to these crass antics were purely experimental and not the last of such efforts, but more of that later when I write of my worst hospital experience. On the bruising experiment being reported to Parry-Williams a letter was sent to Bizzaro telling him not to do anything like that again.

After one particularly violent knee bleed Bizzaro insisted on a caliper or leg brace, irons colloquially, it was fitted in the clinic in the afternoon, I wore it until we reached home when I took it off and threw it in the coal-house. Mum and Dad left it there hoping to persuade me when my temper had subsided and a night's sleep had rendered me as biddable as ever I got. To my delight the coalman paid his monthly visit very early the next day and before he could be stopped dumped a few hundredweight of coal on the offending object. Mum said 'however are we going to get it out' Dad said 'leave it' and gave me a wry smile. When almost all the coal had gone up in smoke Mum told me I'd have to wear it, as soon as she could dig it out, as an appointment with Bizzaro was due. This was a battle I intended to win by agreeing to wear the encumbrance just before the appointed time, in the event my planning proved unnecessary. For lo, it came to pass that when we were out for a walk over the fields more coal was delivered and Bizzaro had to be faced caliper-less. He wasn't angry, astonished and blustering yes, but too shocked for anger, his bald and domed head shaking from side to side and his eyes popping out. 'Under the coal, what, why, I don't understand, couldn't you retrieve it?' Nothing could placate the poor soul and after examining my knee he seemed even more disappointed as no ill effects from my rejection of his contraption had accrued and he dismissed me with a further six-month appointment.

I spent a great deal of time on Sage, the children's ward of Gulson Road Hospital, between the ages of around eighteen months until twelve years; included in that were two Christmas stints when rules were relaxed to the extent that they could be without endangering the patients and really we had a very good time although each of us would have preferred to have been at home. Nurses came and went over the years, all of them wonderful and most of them Irish as Matron would recruit a new intake of girls from Ireland every year for training. Those individual Bredas and Kates who I got to know and invariably liked would move on, usually to other wards in the hospital. If I was lucky I would be able to say goodbye but more often they'd have gone when next I was admitted. Friendships with other patients were the same, often fun, sometimes intense but quickly over and never pursued once I returned home; on the couple of occasions when someone tried to keep in touch I quietly refused to respond. The psychology behind my reluctance is unclear to me but I felt the need to keep the two lives as separate as possible.

Sister Shannon, marvellously reliable and infinitely capable, Gwen who helped feed and wash those unable at the time and Mrs Poole the cleaner were the only staff who were there consistently over the years. Gwen would now be called a nursing assistant or something of the kind but back then everyone knew her as Gwen and didn't question her status. Being a teaching hospital the staff moved to other wards regularly but Gwen was always there with a comforting smile and a gentle presence, and I remember her with love and respect as the closest to an angel that I knew. There was one other permanent nurse who worked with the babies and toddlers exclusively and I remember only one incident concerning her. Visitors were not allowed to bring sweets or fruit directly to the children but had to turn them over to a member of staff and these offerings were kept and doled out equally on saucers after dinner each day; it was always interesting to see what your saucer contained, a few orange segments, the inevitable sprig of grapes, a slice of Mars bar or similar, four or five Smarties, toffees, boiled sweets we never knew what to expect. It was a fair and wise system as some children would otherwise have got nothing, and presentation after the main meal meant no spoiled appetite but it was resented in some quarters and smuggling was resorted to on occasion.

Chapter 2

Mum took a sly look about and slipped me a chocolate bar with the instruction, 'Eat it while I'm here, but be careful, don't let Nurse catch you. She's very sharp!' This was very early in my career as a Sage Wardee and I was in a cot and cared for by this nurse. On the next occasion when she was close to me, tucking in the sheets I studied her face intently and found that my mother was right, at last understanding the meaning of sharp and said: My Mummy says you have a sharp nose! The organ was indeed pointed and thin but I felt I'd seen sharper, anyway it was fairly sharp and I thought she might like to know... Such a look she gave me, uncomprehending and disdainful in turn before shrugging and getting on with 'straightening' the cot. I suspect she preferred babies to children who could talk.

Mum warned me I mustn't cry when visiting time was over because if I did they wouldn't let her come to see me ever again. At the end of next visiting time, blinking to stop the tears I told her 'I'm not crying am I Mummy'. I wanted to hold on to her and cry, yes, and fight and scream but knew I had to hold in the tears. I must have believed what she told me, or did I realise that she wouldn't be able to stand it if I cried, it was wrong of her but so understandable, poor damaged woman, two of her infants had died on that very ward previous to my birth. It's no surprise that I thought only I lay under the threat of complete abandonment if I gave way to tears when others could freely cry and sob. My anger, always close to the surface, would boil up when the others cried and called for mummy over and over. I wanted to hurt them and on one occasion did! I had shouted shut-up to no avail so undid the restrainers that were meant to keep us in the cots, clambered over the side and punched one of them several times. The calling and sobbing carried on just the same, no increase in volume or intensity; the despair of the child was almost total so I don't think my unkind act added to it. Nowadays we know that young children do not 'settle' when separated from their mother but rather collapse into a state of despair so deep that grief itself is eventually subdued into lethargic bereavement. No-one came to stop me and I scrambled back into the cot feeling sorry I'd done it and at the same time glad I had, confused, appalled and frightened.

Sage was arranged so that the babies were nearest the entrance then the toddlers then the boys and lastly the girls. After that came the balcony which was a green-painted metal and glass construction similar to a conservatory tacked on to the end wall of the ward. I don't remember being in the babies ward, each of the sections was referred to as a ward, the Toddler's, the Boy's, the Girl's and each separated by a partition made up of glass and timber panels from floor to ceiling with a central gap the size of double-doors, my memories start from the toddler's. To get from entrance to balcony meant passing through each section.

One or two of the many babies that came onto the ward had oxygen tents over the cot, with a green bucket like device fitted to the head, or was it the foot, of the cot with what in my memory seems to be dry-ice in it, anyway something that let out clouds of vapour, and often these cots would have parents sadly gazing into them and Mum told me not to comment as the babies were very poorly. The maternity ward was situated on the ground floor on the same line as Sage and it could well be that the babies in the oxygen tents were premature and brought up from downstairs. In the Toddlers Ward temperatures were taken by getting the child to lie on its side and inserting the thermometer, lubricated with a little petroleum jelly, into the rectum, the rectal method in fact, my memory of this procedure is strong and I remember how one did not move during the time it took for the thermometer to cook but how marvellous it seemed that the other, even younger, ones never sat up and caused themselves injury, it's almost as though instinct told them to be still, as did the nurses. The thermometers themselves had a smaller reservoir of mercury or its equivalent and this was a metallic blue, presumably the small reservoir meant less chance of an accident and the blue colour meant they were never shoved under a patient's tongue but kept strictly for the posterior orifice, it was a joyous day when I graduated to the other thermometers which were placed under the armpit or eventually used orally. Sometimes however, by the time the nurses got to the balcony only blueys were left and humiliatingly I would be asked to roll onto my side, as I got older I'd refuse and be told what a bold boy I was by the Irish nurse and she would have to retrieve and render sterile a silver thermometer before she could carry on. I might have responded that she was a bold girl, just a few years older, in some cases, than me. On the one or two occasions where I couldn't be bothered to argue, the feeling both anally and also of submission was rather pleasant. Not in any sense erotic, but a definite sensual thrill for a child not given to relinquishing control in any sense. For some years after, until sexual awareness and knowledge were complete, I would have dreams where young women placed me on a table and did pleasant though non-specific things to me!

Spelling my name came easily to me very early, as on admission to hospital Mum would have to rehearse it to the nurse taking down my details, thus I could reel it off without difficulty, not that I was often asked to do so it was more of a party-trick. Less pleasant was being carried up the dog-leg stairs on a stretcher, an ambulance driver at each end and me trying not to slide backwards, I knew I wouldn't fall off the stretcher but worried about my head ramming into the ambulance driver at the rear, might he then stumble or lose the rhythm? No lift on Sage, transport to x-ray or operating theatre and back were achieved the same way.

The x-ray department lay at the end of a long ground-floor corridor and the x-ray room itself had a peculiar chemical and rubber smell which made the air one breathed seem artificial, and the cramped semi-darkness, was conducive of unease on entering an alien environment. Over the years the same radiographer took the x-rays and would often require me to put myself into positions that I found uncomfortable to hold for more than a very short time, any delay meant that I would move, quite involuntarily, and the process would have to be repeated. I hated this as it suggested that I had lost control, and it wasted my time and that of the wavy-white-haired radiographer who always, form my first x-ray at Gulson to my last, looked the same, white hair, white coat and pale face from days spent in that gloomy unhealthy seeming room.

My parents had four children, my brother Syd, fourteen years my senior and Walter and Freda both of whom died in infancy. With the benefit of experience I can see that my parents never got over those deaths. The home always had background sadness, a feeling of absence, in the circumstances understandable, and an air of something left unsaid. Under the stairs, in the gloomy depths that scare a child, were two of those monumental stone vases with a metal grid and cup for water and flowers, these bore the names of the brother and sister I'd never known but missed nonetheless, they remained under the stairs throughout my childhood and early manhood right up until I left home, never mentioned and never touched and whenever I caught sight of them it reinforced my apprehension of death and separation. Tears formed by empathy filled my eyes in those early years but never fell, I knew better than to cry. What happened to the vases when my parents moved away to Cornwall after I left home I never felt able to ask.

How hard for my parents to face the loss of two infant children, Freda aged just twelve months from meningitis, and five years later, Walter aged two years from subarachnoid haemorrhage only to have your next child diagnosed with haemophilia, how hard to have your doctor promise an early death for this last born child.

An unfortunate consequence of my diagnosis is that Doctor Vaughn refused to keep me as a patient, claiming, according to my mother, that 'they die before they reach fourteen and I don't want the responsibility.' Mum and I moved on to Doctor Mellor who always did the little he could for my condition with great patience and promptness, providing adequate pain relief, vitamin K (Kapilon tablets) vital in the clotting process and, as I didn't eat well, a sensible precaution, and wintergreen ointment for bruising. A quick decision would be taken and he would send me off to Harry Parry when unsure.

Very often my bleeds were not treated any better in hospital, the pain control was much worse and no factor replacement existed, occasionally I received plasma or whole blood but this was by no means invariable and up until I was about twelve years old I could count and indeed point to the sites where intravenous drips had been administered. In fairness I have to add that my mother denied this, telling me I'd had 'transfusions' every time I'd been admitted, but being on the receiving end of the procedure I definitely know better! I had heard it said, too many times and at too young an age, that the family doctor had refused me as a patient on my finally receiving a diagnosis, predicting an early demise.

I knew death. I had already been too close to it on a couple of occasions. Once, when the faces and attitudes told me that matters were very serious, I was given a drip of plasma, which was rare in itself. This may have been when I had received a blow in the throat from another boy at Corley Open Air School and bled into the tissues and down the throat into the stomach too, but I think it was even further in the past before I started school. The other time the drip was taken down by Doctor Scott who was, I now assume, one of Mr Parry-Williams' S H O's. At that age whenever I had a drip set up my arm would be immobilised on a splint with bandaging. Doctor Scott started to cut the bandaging with scissors and unfortunately began to cut me as well. Although it hurt I hadn't the strength to struggle and could only protest: You're cutting me! He withdrew the scissors and said 'No Derek, I'm only cutting the bandage, I'd never do anything to hurt you'.

Chapter3

As the bandage came away he leant forward and then looked me in the eyes with a stricken expression and admitted the truth: Oh, Derek I'm so sorry - I have cut you!

The cut was small, not deep and only a few millimetres long so didn't of itself give me any further problem. I must have been very weak as I didn't even flinch and the measure of love and trust I felt prevented the cursing and swearing which was my usual defence and of which I was an adept. Doctor Scott was a special man and a friend, often lifting me up to touch the ceiling which seemed so high and remains so in my memory, he must have been particularly tall. What a team Harry Parry-Williams had in those early days, and incidentally what an N.H.S. we had in its early days, the other team members were female, Doctors Ingram and Gaffney both highly competent and lovely people. Doctor Gaffney was I suspect his registrar, more about her when I write about school. I felt loved and valued by these people, as any child ought to expect, and safe in their hands. I believed that all of us were determined to see that I did not die before the age of fourteen and decided that when I reached that age I would go to see the G.P. who'd signed so many death certificates of family members and crow over him. When I reached my fourteenth birthday my mother forbade me as 'He's an old man now, and it wouldn't be fair. I know what you're like.' I protested but it was only the prompting of my reputation as I was secretly glad having other things to do and anyway it was only the promise to self that was driving me, besides it would be tempting fate...... The thing that I detested on the Toddlers were restrainers, a sort of vest that opened down the back, and had two straps of the same material, which would be put on under the pyjama jacket and tied with a bow to the bars at the back of the cot, this meant that while it was possible to sit up, lie down and turn onto a side it was impossible to run up and down the cot or climb and fall out. I resented this interference most strongly and quickly learned how to undo the bow by feel as it was of course impossible to see it. By this method I could maintain independence until the next time the bed was made and, when no-one was looking, run up and down the cot or climb over the side to the floor and back up again. The nurses would sometimes tie a double bow and that took a bit more patience to undo, and occasionally they would tie intricate knots which took even longer, and, if left alone by me, irritated the next set of bed-making nurses. On occasion other kids got loose but this would be down to an incompetently or hurried bow-tying, one little boy was required to give a specimen of urine and was so young that he was still in nappies;

when this was the case the bemused child would have a medicine bottle taped to his penis until the necessary specimen was produced. This boy got free of the restrainers stood up and charged up and down the cot with the medicine bottle swinging and banging off each fat little thigh and his penis stretched to the limit. He was unconcerned and happy, a big grin on his face as though he were about to win his country a medal. It amused me so much that I hoped it would go on forever, but the truth was that the bottle would have worked loose and possibly smashed on the parquet floor. All too soon two nurses hurried across: Ahh Breda, would you look at the cut of him! Poor child, and you Derek Haughton, you bold boy, don't be laughing like that. But they were holding back their own mirth, and I knew it.

Soon enough the message got through that no restrainers could hold me and the whole idea was dropped, apart from the odd nurse new to the ward and who'd been told all the toddlers were to be restrained. I would refuse the damned things and the nurse would check and that would be the end of the matter, and not long after I graduated to the Boys Ward. One last memory of my time in the Toddlers Ward was being required to remain there, when I had no bleed and felt well, for a series of daily intramuscular injections in the thigh, these were painful and were administered daily for perhaps a fortnight, causing immense bruising all over the thighs, purple and mauve, hot and painful to the touch. All through my childhood and early teens I had many blood tests and heard discussions around the subject of a low blood count, Parry-Williams would say that he knew all about my low blood-count and that everything had been tried to raise it but an initial response was never maintained, were these injections one of the things that had been tried, also the transfusions of whole blood? Whatever the cause of the anomaly it disappeared eventually and hasn't been mentioned once since adulthood but was the reason I had to spend a few days more in Birmingham General after a tooth extraction in my early teens. A blood test led to me being asked if I had a bleed, then the next day was I sure I hadn't a bleed and on the third day being told I must be honest, was there blood in my urine or faeces. I insisted there was not and at last the problem was explained to me, when I asked them to phone Parry-Williams who would explain, this done I was allowed home.

Shortly after this painful imposition I graduated to the boys ward. To be trusted in a bed and to be with older boys was to be promoted to undreamed of heights. I could now disobey the rules and get out of bed to pass something across the ward to another; this was usually undertaken when the several nurses went to 'break' as the odds were then tipped in my favour. A girl Barbara whose name I have never forgotten and who attended Baginton Fields school later in both our lives asked me to get her water from the sink next to the bed I occupied on that admission, she smiled at me and as I had been susceptible to the charms of a pretty face ever since my first noticing girls, I did it. She snatched the water from me and never smiled at me again, then or later when we attended the same school. Other lessons could be physically painful, the boy in the next bed, seemed a good friend but when we were playing with toy cars on the locker which separated the beds suddenly leant forward and with both hands dug his nails into my neck, with a maniacal look on his face, pulled his hands back and left four throbbing red wheals on each side. My neck remained sore to the touch for a couple of days. Authority was unaware and that's the way it stayed, to tell would have broken the code by which we lived. I never even acknowledged his existence from that moment however, despite his pleas to talk and play with him. He had rendered himself an unstable character dangerous to me, so only fit to be ignored. Other boys became great friends for a while, but these alliances and friendships lasted only as long as the 'gang' were together on the ward, the same thing happened with members of staff, one would look forward to a particular favourite coming on duty, but they always moved on to other wards and that meant in most cases goodbye. The odd thing is that I have in my mind's eye just one boy from those times, not that our friendship was prolonged, he came and went so quickly back to his usual life, and others had spent longer on the ward with me but I remember nothing of them. This is not strictly true as far as other haemophiliacs were concerned, there was a core of us who met up regularly, Michael, Tony, Brian and I, all around the same age and a younger boy or two whose haemophilia was only mild to moderate. I was introduced to the grandfather of one of these boys, presumably as a form of encouragement, a man in his early sixties also a haemophiliac, such encouragement was unnecessary as I already knew I was not going to die young.

When death took a child screens were erected down the middle of the boys and girls wards on each side to form a corridor and a trolley would be wheeled down carrying the deceased, further hidden by a leather contrivance pulled up into place by the porters. As soon as the screens came out I knew what was happening and as a very young boy soon apprised my more innocent although curious companions of the facts. Later I learned not to say anything as it always led to an unseemly fuss with kids jumping up and down on their beds trying to see and pulling at the screens.

One night on being awoken by unusual activity, I had seen through the partition a child being washed all over and then wrapped in what seemed to me to be metre on metre of bandaging. The child was obviously dead because nobody ever got bathed in the night and the only movement came when they lifted an arm or leg, the nurses were not sharing a quiet chat but were solemn faced and silent. I was sorry that it had happened, although this was a toddler I didn't know, but I was glad I had learned a little more about death and its aftermath.

So I lived my life with the knowledge of death and often found trouble by making sure that I wasn't the only child so burdened.

Chapter 4

One wretched boy told another 'Your daddy's older than mine; your daddy's going to die.' I detested the gloating way this was said and decided to give him the benefit of my knowledge, I told him everyone's going to die. 'No they're not.' 'Yes they are' I told him. 'Not my Mummy and Daddy?' 'Yes.' 'Not me?' 'Yes, and it doesn't matter how old people are, that's got nothing to do with it!' He shut up.

Most of these kids were extremely raw when it came to the facts of existence and hardly one of them had been in hospital before. I on the other hand had been on the ward many times and knew the ropes, what could and could not be got away with for instance. I also learned to recognise appendicitis cases on admission by the way they walked slightly bent over supporting the lower abdomen, obviously in pain. One of these bods on my telling him he very likely would be having his appendix out told me I was stupid and the doctor was only going to look at him, give him medicine and then he could go home. I resented his impudence, 'The doctor will come, he'll examine you but he won't have any medicine and will shove his finger up your bum.' 'No, he won't, don't be dirty. I'm telling.' At this point I could see the SHO and a nurse coming up the ward with a trolley. 'Here's the doctor now.' Screens around the bed, 'Lie on your left side, that's right now pull up your knees and relax.' a yell of outraged disbelief and a sharp command to keep still, then quiet, the screens removed, distressed bod looks at me and sobs, reluctantly acknowledging the ward's fount of all knowledge.

I very soon enhanced that reputation and renewed it on every admission. By the use of a trick learned by observation I would be able to tell the boys whether or not they were going home after the eagerly awaited Harry Parry ward round. Someone would be convinced they were going home but I knew better, or someone would be cast down because they thought they were not going home, I knew better! This trick was so mysterious that I would be asked after H.P. and his entourage had moved on, am I going home, what about me etc. Some would get a definite yes others a no, and others I would say that it was unclear. At every bed there would be an examination and a review of tests and x-rays where applicable and if the decision was that a boy was to be discharged then a pink slip would be written out and paper-clipped to the notes. I would manage to see this unless the position of the entourage blocked my view. When first I showed my superior knowledge I would be jeered but after being proved right I had it made as a fortune teller.

The cocky boy so ready to tell another that his father was going to die kept silent until visiting time was almost over then complained to his parents thus conferring a kind of pariah status upon himself. We didn't like that sort of thing. Sister was sent for and the incensed father pointed at me and yelled 'he told my son he was going to die.' Sister asked if it was true, I didn't explain the circumstances but said: I told the truth, everyone is going to die. The father jumped up and shouted 'He's saying it again, he's saying it again! Which was also the truth, indeed I was. I don't remember the outcome but I'm sure I would not have retracted.

When at home, on occasion only briefly, I was the complete suburban boy which fact I look back on with gratitude; in the country I would, most probably not have survived, being further away from medical care and on streets enclosed by other streets would not have had half the fun. Immediately at the back of my house was the cratered and rubble-strewn expanse known to us kids as The Dump or The Tip, to most parents an eyesore but paradise to us, and beyond that another field always known as The Cornfield and then field after field, lane after lane, swamp and flood and river.

Unless taken for a walk we younger children never went further than Dump and Cornfield but these, when slightly older, were the open-range, the rolling sea, battle-ground and homeland.

The more domestically oriented of the little girls utilised the house bricks that littered the terrain by laying them end to end to represent walls with gaps for doors, and simulated family life. A solitary boy would be collared as the father, or if very young the baby, and be ordered and chivvied about until the other boys arrived and he could join the cowboys, Indians, pirates and soldiers roaming at will, shooting and stabbing, hacking and chopping, havocking and pillaging, dying and rising again, imagination unfettered, wild and careless. As I grew towards five years old I joined in, though not quite so fearlessly.

I spent the first three years of my education at a residential school so am able to separate my childhood into three discrete sections very easily. Three years away didn't bother me at all, I was used to being away from home after many in-patient visits to hospital and able to find my feet at once in any situation, having suffered very little deliberate unkindness from children and none at all from the adults I'd met. Inevitably this was to change, but those years before school were, on looking back, very good times and the bad times not so very bad at all, apart from the physical pain of bleeding into knees and elbows and the emotional pain of enforced, repeated separation on admission to hospital.

Mum singing as she worked, the crack and snap of the sheets on the washing line, the questing sound of a small plane flying high but under the sailing clouds, the soft noises the hens made as they foraged in the litter, the calling of birds these meant home.

Our mid-terrace, two bed roomed house was, at that time, rented and had been completed in a hurry just before the war when all building of homes stopped for the duration. Grandad painted the rooms with distemper, each room a different colour with a stippled finish and strips of dado paper above, and the ceilings whitened. The internal doors were all grained by him, a brown colour applied over cream and then manipulated with 'combs' to look like natural wood, I doubt my memory as far as colour goes and I only know he did it because I was told, but the décor remained the same until I reached the age of around eleven years.

My first memory of Grandad is looking up at him and marvelling at the size of his belly as he sat reading the paper by the fire, and knowing he didn't want to be disturbed. His dog, Billy, also hugged the fire and crawling over to him on the coconut matting, I must have been very young, I reached out for his tail, Grandad warned 'He'll snap you', I took no notice pulling back my hand as he 'snapped' me.

My Dad called Billy, Pink Eye because he had an area of pink skin around one eye, his more interesting possession was a lump of sulphur yellow stuff in his drinking bowl, to keep him healthy I was told and I always envied it trying to sneak a bite but never succeeded.

When Mum and I left for home he would follow the pushchair and Mum would turn round and tell him to go home, off he'd trot back the way we had come but turn up an alley and a couple of hundred yards further on would appear again just behind us, and I, straining to look behind would chuckle and Mum would again send him back. Sometimes by use of this tactic he would arrive at our door simultaneous with our own arrival and would then be sent back. I would beg that he be allowed to come in but Mum always correctly said no as he'd do it every day and might have an accident. He was a very sensible dog in a number of ways, although he 'snapped' me he took care to miss, was adept at crossing roads alone, and although often aggressive to others of his kind, would fight only those no bigger than himself, if a big dog came up the street he would cross to the other side and then cross back over when the larger dog had gone on its way.

When Grandad broke his leg he bought, to assist him with his recovery, an inflatable red rubber doughnut like ring to take the weight off his backside as he had to sit so much. On his return to full mobility this lived under the cushion on the easy chair in the corner of the living-room, on my lifting the cushion to get a look at this enticing rubber construction Gran would say leave that it's Grandad's. I longed for him to get it out so that I could see it inflated and maybe taken to where we could use it together and have a wonderful time. He never even looked at it as I would have done were it mine, instead it languished far from the element where it's fabulous nature could have been seen and utilised. One day I could stand it no longer; he chuckled and rumpled my hair before showing it to me. Interrupting his perusal of the paper and misunderstanding the nature of the object I'd said: Grandad! When are you going to get your rubber dinghy out?

Grandad gave me my first taste of beer when we were in the garden of the local pub, the Devonshire Arms, I must have been three or four years old when he leant forward on the bench and held his glass to my lips 'Here have a taste.' I took a sip and remember the bitterness and spitting it out to hear his laughter. You may think this an unusual and wrong thing for an adult to do to a child but I assure you that this was a trick played widely on the young in those days. The other treat he brought for me was much more to my taste and he would sit me up on the table and run his hand up and down my back and call me Billy Square Back, and say when you grow up you'll be a good 'un, then he would produce a Crunchie bar from his pocket, present it and chuckle. Always a Crunchie bar and Gran always gave me a Mars bar, I see now that these were part of their ration, the austerity still in force included rationing of sweets.

I imagine the redecorating took place once Dad bought the property from the landlord. The consistent nature of the fabric of home helped to mitigate the insecurity as love, anger and confusion fought for supremacy on repeated admissions to hospital, the décor the entire fabric of house and garden, and favourite items of furniture too.

Chapter 5

In what was known as the front room lived (there are no inanimate objects in the life of a young child) two of my favourite beings, an upright piano and The Bureau always given the reverence of spoken initial capitals befitting its status as the repository of important papers, sparse family archives, old letters arbitrarily kept as significant, a mass of old photographs in one of the drawers and Mum's gold watch. This watch was reputed to be broken, over-wound by a young female relative who borrowed it to wear on a night out; thirty years later it turned out that all it needed was a clean by a watch repairer and then kept perfect time.

The Bureau fascinated me for if you lowered the writing surface front, two brackets, the upper surfaces of which were covered with green baize, magically emerged from as supports. Lowering and raising the writing surface and lid was a surreptitious delight watching these supports emerge and retract to faceted square decorations over and over again, if noticed I'd be told to come away as I must never 'go in' The Bureau and besides I might catch my fingers in the metal stays that prevented too much weight going onto the supports.

The piano was never tuned and hardly ever played, occasionally Dad could be persuaded, at Christmas or when my brother and sister-in-law visited, to give us a tune but he accomplished this by ear playing only on the 'black notes'. I never saw him dance but here was a man full of song and recitation, a performer frustrated by the necessity of earning a living according to the conventions of his life and times.

I wish I was a navvy
Working on the line
Four and twenty bob a week
And working overtime.

Dad, when in a particularly good mood, gave forth rhyme and song and monologue mostly learned from the music halls he delighted in when young but he could also slip into deep melancholy, controlled but evident to an observant child.

Past tragic circumstance played a part in his sadness for he struggled to come to terms with the loss of the two infants prior to my birth and the recent death of his sister Win.

Mostly he was a cheerful man, at least in my presence, though unpredictable at times and much given, as I, to sudden fits of singing and acting. Some of his rhymes and jokes I never got to hear all the way through as my mother would interject to stop him: Syddddd, don't! He knows enough stuff of that sort already, for instance:

There was a young lady
From Amsterdam
Who cocked her leg over
A pot of jam......................Sydddd don't!

Another partial lyric based on a song from the North-East was:

As I was going to Sandgate
To Sandgate, to Sandgate
As I was going to Sandgate
I met a dirty wench..........

Again Mum's protesting voice was heard, as familiar, necessary and ultimately boring as the talk of big-ends, tappets and differential gear boxes that plagued the ears of a child born into a city heavily involved in producing motor cars. If Dad and I were alone he exercised his internal censor so maybe he set out to tease Mum with his revelatory and lubricious warbling and uttering, you get the picture, no need for more of his rhymes about less than ladylike young ladies or people taken short on corridor free trains. Other verbal spasms were more acceptable and indeed Mum would sometimes join in; it was a pleasure to hear their duet. Near the mark but not quite over it:

...................Nelly so fat
Dressed up like an acrobat

When she tried to do the splits
The copper put out the lights.......

It ended there so whatever happened next in the song I never found out! Curiously these next two were never subject to Mum's censoring:

Once upon a time
When there was no lime
And the bricklayers had no mortar
There came a little bird
And he dropped a little turd
And the bricklayers had some mortar.

And to the tune of the British Grenadiers:

There was a bonny Scotsman
And he came to Waterloo
The wind blew up his trouser leg
And tickled his cock-a-doodle-oo.

A rhyming couplet went: seven and six I paid to be wed, I wish I'd bought a bulldog instead. This, a reference to the fact that both dog licence and marriage licence cost exactly the same, seven shillings and six pence, this provided me an explanation why so many married women led what seemed to me a dog's life and were often compelled to consort with vicars to the detriment of such, according to the News of the World, presumably as payback for clergy officiating at their ultimately corrosive weddings.

My most cherished memories of Dad come from childhood Sunday mornings. He'd read the newspapers in bed and I'd join him, if it was a cold morning he would invariably say Snoogle Mcdougal and grin as I buried myself under the covers, mum would bring us both a cup of tea and he'd give me the picture paper to 'read'. I'd examine the pictures, and once capable of reading get what I could from the captions then switch to the other paper, there were always three, and read the few stories that appealed to me, pretty soon Dad would have finished the scurrilous News of the World and hover expectantly, never actually taking the paper I was reading but looking me in the face and waiting for me to finish the sentence I was reading, his hand twitching. We'd then exchange papers and I would marvel at yet another vicar being defrocked for inappropriate behaviour with a parishioner, usually a married woman, though what exactly the reverent gentlemen had done I had no idea, if I asked Dad he would say 'He behaved like a bit of a rat.' or shake his head which meant either I don't know or I don't wish to comment. I marvelled that the supply of rodent like clergymen never seemed to diminish and that so many married women were prepared to join them in whatever frowned-upon activity they instigated.

Reading done, Dad would sing to me, try as I might I cannot recall most of what he sang but some remains, a good deal concerning the sea.

Barnacle Bill the sailor, though not much of that as I fear it contained lyrics Mum would not have approved of. Another song had the line, the captain took his whiskers off and fried them for his tea, a curious image and that explains why I remember it. The gallant Captain Billy

Brown who played his ukulele as the ship went down won my admiration every time. My Bonny Lies Over The Ocean was a big favourite which because of my peculiar habit of insisting that my baby sun hat was a bonnet (most of my fellow toddlers were girls) insinuated into my mind a sad image, which I still recall, of my sun hat floating out to sea. Three songs I recall a little more of are these.

Poor Joe.

A carriage rolled by
With a lady inside
She looked on poor Joe
As her own darling child
She gave him a penny
To buy him some bread
And although he was singing
He wished himself dead.

I well understood the last words as when in severe pain I often felt tempted to wish the same; I never did as I knew I'd feel differently when the pain subsided. What I didn't understand was the insouciance of the lady in the carriage, again I misread the situation and the image conjured was of a carriage crashing and tumbling over and over down the hill. The lady in peril of her life could still concentrate enough to think of poor Joe and somehow give him a penny when she must have been rattling around inside the rolling carriage. Such bravery never failed to bring tears and Dad would cheer me up with this.

The preamble, or as much as I remember: This old moke somehow or other's been to me just like a brother.....

Up at Bed'orth on holiday
He earned me piles o' quids
Till all the dirty kids started,
Hangin' on behind
Hangin' on behind.
Pulling all his horse hair out
Till my poor bony lookin' nag
Didn't have a little bit of tail to wag
So I supplied a new one
Bearing mind, now he
Waggles a razor-strap
With a toothbrush
Hangin' on behind.

I think both of us were saddened when the Sunday morning ritual came to an end.

Not that the fun did. His sudden bursts of facetiousness could still delight, mostly because of his obvious pleasure in what he sang, said or did. He would burst forth with: Oh, go to Joan Glover and tell her I love her. This would be followed by a wheezing chuckle and a grin, he obviously believed that I knew this from school as it usually appeared when that place was mentioned, and the chuckle would be accompanied by a conspiratorial look, puzzling but which seemed to imply something like 'I know you find this as ridiculous as I.' I had however never heard of the thing and this remained true until just a few years ago when I heard the round, Joan Glover, sung on television and after all the intervening years Dad's certainty that I would find it ludicrous lost its mystery.

More or less vulgar, depending on your interpretation of vulgar, were the comments elicited by audible flatulence, these consisted of two possibilities: Let go the painter! Or Trumpeter What Are You Sounding Now? The first of these a continuation of the nautical theme in a number of his songs, the second from words written by J. Francis Barron to the tune by J. Airlie Dix published 1904. Because my own vulgarity has proved fireproof and survived the blasts of super-heated hot-air fired, orifice unnamed, by many an authority, I reproduce here the first few lines of the song, bearing in mind Dad's novel usage.

Trumpeter, what are you sounding now?
(Is it the call I'm seeking?)
'You'll know the call,' said the Trumpeter tall,
'When my trumpet goes a speakin'.

The piano had curious square section 'legs' between the keyboard and its feet and these rather than supporting anything could be spun round , I would crawl under the keyboard and sit pressing the pedals and reaching up into its innards to play notes from underneath to Mum's accompaniment of 'mind you don't get your fingers stuck'. All the years we owned the piano I never felt stimulated to try for a more conventional approach to coaxing out the music it concealed.

Chapter 6

Her father dead at seven and orphaned, on her mother's death, at thirteen, Mum suffered the loss of two infants, and lived through the blitz only to be told that her youngest son was to die before the age of fourteen, that she found the knowledge difficult to live with is surely a given, that she remained sane is a wonder and a witness to her resilience and stubborn nature. Her belief in the doctor's prediction is not strange as doctors were looked on as minor gods, as was anyone with more than an elementary education. Perhaps when she'd known a few more representatives of the species, as I suffered bleed after bleed, she came to amend her view.

She first noticed swollen fingers where I'd caught them in my shawl, as babies will but the real problems started when I learned to crawl and developed my first knee bleed, I dare say I cried and was impossible to settle and she must have been worried that this was another doomed child.

On my eventual diagnosis she became my escort to many a clinic and, unfortunately, the one who signed me in to many an in-patient ordeal of separation. This had to be done and I acknowledge it but at the time I felt it as a betrayal and would fight against it but the love she gave was unconditional and never stinted even when I began to attack her both verbally and physically. Her patience, loving care and understanding of the dynamics of the situation were heroic. I regret the pain I caused her, from my diagnosis until the age of around three or four, and admit that it took me years to regain control of my temper but mostly I regret that, even toward the end of her life, she was the one person who could rile me into fury and my consolation is that the depth of my feeling for her drove the anger. I knew that she understood. One day as I engaged in biting, scratching or pulling her hair, in spite of the pain she sang under her breath, 'You always hurt the one you love.' I wish I could write here that I desisted at that point but remember, even now, how being found out only added to my fury.

For years I lived with the conflict of self-criticism and disgust on the one hand and easily aroused anger on the other. Any misunderstanding or perceived slight, especially from friends or loved ones, would provoke outright rage, a feeling I learned to control only through great struggle and which is now reduced to ash and embers. I have come to understand the terrible time Mum and I went through and no longer heap blame on either head but know that my response was one of a number of possible responses to an unbearable situation for a child. Now I feel only compassion for a little boy facing rejection over and over, and a doting mother, hurt by so much death in her life and wonder how things might have been without stubbornness and determination on both sides. I suspect the outcome could have been fatal for at least one of them.

The living-room contained the usual compliment of furniture including dining table and chairs and in a large alcove kitchen area with cooker, sink, a 'copper' for the weekly wash, and I suppose although I have no memory of them a few shelves. Once in the alcove it was possible to gaze into the space under the stairs where the electricity and gas meters dwelt and further into the gloom the two sad and chilling stone monumental vases, spiders and who knows what. To the right of the alcove a separate door led into the pantry, a four foot square floor space and many shelves with a large cold slab which formed the roof of the outside coal shed next to the back door the coal shed being about four foot square with its own door.

Upstairs there were two bedrooms and a bathroom/ WC. The front bedroom was my parents, mine too as before Corley I slept in the same room, and the back bedroom accommodated Syd.

The furniture in the front bedroom was beautiful, with its walnut panels cut to make full use of the grain, and had been bought second-hand off a Jewish couple from just over the road on their emigrating to Israel after the war. The large wardrobe had a door made up of three panels so arranged as to look, to me at least, like a river emerging from a cave and pouring down as a waterfall, I loved this scene whether or not others saw it in the same way I don't know.

Before I went to Corley Dad constructed a sort of conservatory around the back door and coal house, this had an asbestos sheet roof and lots of glass, also a section of the floor was cobbled with large pebbles set in cement, why that should be I don't know, it was only one corner, a corner I very quickly learned to avoid as it was so easy to turn my ankle and I really didn't want an ankle bleed. I have a strong impression that the outhouse as it was called was used on wash day and that the copper was installed out there, this seems unlikely however as a gas supply would have been needed, surely a long piece of tubing from the kitchen alcove and out of the open back door could not have been utilised? Perhaps the intention was spoken about and my memory comes from that. I have no recollection of anything else out there, so what its function was meant to be is beyond me.

Dad also constructed the garage at the end of the garden; this building was made with corrugated iron sides, an asbestos roof, and full-length windows across the front facing the house, double doors facing the entry and another door from the garden path. The only part of this structure I actually remember him creating was the floor made of house bricks, I recall him taking me in through the smaller door and showing me the floor whilst telling me it would now be possible to sleep in the garage, of course I asked him when we could do so and he chuckled and ruffled my hair but I hoped that one day his suggestion would be made fact and anticipated it with excitement mixed with some trepidation concerning the unfamiliar.

My pedal-car was kept in the garage, an appropriate venue, handy for 'driving' it out into the entry and up and down a short way though I very soon learned to ignore its allure as on two occasions unknown to anyone but me my foot slipped off the pedal and catching on the ground my leg was pulled back under the seat, perhaps this caused a bleed, all I know is when it happened again in spite of taking great care, I reluctantly decided never to get in the thing again and never did.

These memories from very early in my life, when I was small, occur against a background of most people, and everything else, seeming very tall, especially the back gate which was constructed out of chestnut palings nailed to a frame, any chestnut palings I've seen since have been no more than four foot high but the gate I see in my mind is over six feet!

Dad had kept fowl as a boy and constructed a warm, safe and sturdy hen house, rat proof with proper nest boxes and a wire-netting run. There was a smaller house for a broody hen and, later, her chicks, with a door, a window of 'pimply' glass for light and a popping-hole at the side. This shed played a big part in my life as even after the hens and their home were long gone it remained. Dad kept a record of egg production, and those hens really did produce, during rationing eggs could be swapped for other rationed goods and this made catering much easier. The small eggs from the pullets were mine, so Mum told me, little eggs specially laid by the new hens for their little boy. Boiled eggs never tasted better.

I ate very little in fact, if not suffering from a bleed into knee or elbow joint I'd be recovering from the same and if fit and well had no time to waste on inessentials like food. One thing I did long to try was strictly for the birds, Carswood Chicken Spice.

Chapter 7

The chicken spice, a rusty red exotic meal, was a weekly addition to the chicken feed and had, to me at least, a mouth-watering odour but Mum always managed to prevent my attempts at experimental ingestion. Now this was strange as she hardly ever caught me at other pantry misdeeds. Sugar remained on ration (I still have a couple of family ration books) and my unlawful and ultimately disappointing trick was to misappropriate saccharin tablets and suck the sweetness until, in their way, they turned nasty and then spit them out onto the pantry floor, only once did my mother notice them. I was in many ways a wilful, wild and determined child and physical punishment being forbidden I merely had to endure disapproval and mild censure for as long as it took to be over. If I could outlast pain then I could outlast any sanction, besides, I was cute! In my defence, as far as the saccharin tabs were concerned, confectionary being on ration I craved the comfort of sweet things, although born during rationing I knew the lure of the paper-bag and the crinkly wrapper. I suppose most of the sweet ration went to me as my brother was so much older.

I had a little friend named Elizabeth, born in Scotland, she and her parents lived just a few houses down the street, she would come to the back gate and ask 'Can I play in your wee, little hoose?' Elizabeth had a charmingly gentle voice, this and her accent duly charmed me and for the next few years I referred to her as my girlfriend. We spent quite a few hours in that little chicken shed playing house and she showed me how to construct a table out of two picture books, one standing upright half-open for table legs and the other flat as table top. We and her dolls and my teddies feasted many times at that table. The books into table trick I demonstrated to anyone who was prepared to watch.

Other friends shared my 'wee little hoose' occasionally and it served us boys as den, cave or fort until it disappeared during one of my hospital stays. My mother may have insisted on its removal after the Twins, Ronnie and I filled it with ripe wheat, taken by the armful, from The Cornfield in what was probably its last year as a cornfield. Yes, at that time Wyken was suburbia indeed! Mum was angry and frightened and insisted we take it back.

Once the 'wee little hoose' was gone, my playhouse became an asbestos sheet contraption built by Syd to enclose a target for his air-rifle, this had a roof and sides to catch any ricochets and an open front and when not in use I would take my stuffed toys in there to be lined up and admonished as to their future behaviour, treated for any 'bleeds' and fed. Left in there when something else caught my attention, they met their doom and I avoided mine as that night I was removed once more into hospital. On returning home some time later that month the first thing I noticed was that a collapse of my 'cave' had taken place and the remains of my toys were rain sodden and squashed, the elephant's stuffing strewn around, the koala and a couple of others ruined beyond all hope, the only survivor being Ted who by chance had been protected from the rain though squashed and so my favourite teddy bear was resurrected and thereafter accompanied me everywhere I found myself banished to.

My distress and anger at my parents for allowing the disaster can be imagined, and to leave my animal friends to rot in the rain was a betrayal of us all. Of course I blamed myself too, for leaving them out and trusting that all would be well as my parents would look after them.

My other friends were Brian, who lived next door, Ronnie a few houses further along, Angela, Jim who lived a few streets away and Billy, who had a sister, Carol, and lived in the next street. Billy died one Christmas when we were on the same ward in the same hospital, I have no idea what illness brought about his demise, as previously he'd seemed without health problems. Twice I spent Christmas on that ward, once before beginning school so I must have been under five when Billy died.

On Boxing Day a pantomime was performed by the staff on a stage in the hall of the nurses home attached to the hospital. All the patients who could be moved from the wards were taken there by wheelchair stretcher or trolley, only the sickest being left on the wards. Billy did not come to the panto and a few days later he died. I found it hard to accept Billy's death as he had seemed so healthy until his final illness, whatever it was, and besides I was the one supposed to die.

I'd been pleased to have Billy on the ward as he represented home and besides it showed that I was not so unusual if he could end up ill enough to warrant a spell of hospital care. Although I knew he was quite ill I looked forward to his getting better, hoping we'd be on the mend at the same time and could have some fun before we both left for home. When he didn't make it to the panto I knew his condition was very serious, I can't honestly say whether he died while I remained on the ward or after I left for home, my feeling is that I awoke one morning to find him gone.

On another Christmas day, mid-afternoon, I was put on a trolley and pushed around the various wards where the nurses got me to sing and tell jokes. This admission took place from my residential school. A few tut-tuttings were evident from the more outraged but I think the majority were delighted by one so young having the temerity to tell such jokes complete with humorous misquotes as I tried to make sense of the content. The songs always met with approval all round. Even the nurses were mildly put out by my jokes, the older ones would ask me to tell them a joke hoping to scandalise their younger fellows who had been recruited, in a great many cases from Roman Catholic schools in Ireland where matron used to look for a new intake every year. 'Ah, you're a bold boy, however did you get so bold and you so young, Derek Haughton?' The answer was that I had been sent off to school at the age of five and had also spent many days in hospital but this is in retrospect, at the time wherever I happened to be was my life, which never seemed extraordinary and exposed me to many different people, old and young, cultured and vulgar, and what I learned, I learned.

Christmas on the ward was made as happy a time as possible, decorations were put up by the nurses and on one of my Christmas 'visits' the windowsills were covered in a cream, made of what I don't know, which was whipped up and spread like snow and the Christmas tree was decorated with lights that looked like test tubes each filled with a different coloured fluid with a bubble moving from top to bottom of each, a startling and quite beautiful effect never to be seen again. I discovered a photograph of this tree in Mum's papers, too dark and the lights as described not clearly seen but nothing there to tarnish my memory.

The normal rules were suspended and those of us on bed-rest got up after lights out for a bit of fun, which on this occasion involved removal of pyjamas and tying two large handkerchiefs together around the waist as loincloths then running into the girls ward and dancing round and round, with savage gestures and wild ululating, the lamp that lowered down to a couple of feet above the floor.

One boy pretended to be asleep as he was afraid of getting into trouble. Small boys are by nature intolerant of a 'goody-goody' and we surrounded his bed after the war dance was over, not one of us believed him to be asleep and so he was shaken, slapped lightly, poked with a ruler, his feet were tickled with a feather and when none of this produced his 'awakening' his hands and feet were tied up with sticky tape and a jug or two of water poured over him. He was left to shout for help as we all got back into bed, but he remained silent until discovered by a nurse making a round of all the beds. This was bullying, no mistake, though it could have been brought to an end after the first shake of his shoulder, he would not have been believed but could have faked just waking when nothing more than noises of disgust would have been heard. I felt that we should not have done it, but understood why we had and also felt admiration for the fact that he stuck to a course of action once decided on, without complaint and without snitching on those involved.

I remember other boys and girls but not as friends, the lad with diabetes who struggled to come to terms with it and craved sweets. He would pretend that his insulin dosage was too high and fake slipping into a coma to get a Mars Bar or something and when this trick no longer produced the goods, he felt obliged to steal boiled sweets from the cleaner's coats hanging in their locker. He was caught, and although I could never have allowed myself to do such a thing, I felt sorry for him as I could see how difficult he found his diabetes.

A slightly older boy in the next bed to me had a condition that required melted wax to be poured over his shoulder and arm, what good this did I have no idea, what I do recall is that he had lumps under his armpit and that he told me they were caused by acid accumulation, even at the time I was sceptical of his explanation but glad that he was so certain of getting cured by the hot wax that he hated and endured every day. During this same admission a strange girl would leave her bed and run backwards and forwards all over the boys and girls wards on tiptoe, trying to open the windows and when she found one that would open she yelled out of it: What's the time, what's the time? The nurses would grab her and lead her back to bed and sedate her then all would be quiet until the next time, no-one neither children nor staff made a cruel comment or laughed at her, this would not have been the case at another horrible hospital where even the slightest idiosyncrasy or mistake would lead to weeks or months of ridicule from patients and staff alike, but Sage was a good ward in a good hospital with good staff, Dotheboys Hospital was its antithesis. I went home before either of these last cases was resolved and on my next visit they were gone.

Books as I got older would sustain me through many an admission but when younger imaginative play was my usual resort.

Chapter 8

Plasticene, various small toys, comics and later books sustained me after the internal bleeding and pain were subdued, the Plasticene was used to make imaginative adventures concrete and many a sky rocket, or Native American, his tent, arms, campfire and bison he was chasing were constructed on the back of a suitable annual book which acted as a tray. Sometimes it was a log-cabin or a defensive position with a soldier or two, or a re-telling of a story line from a comic, Dangerous Dan's cow pie, or the boy who had a metal fish, a sort of submarine, and met adventure under the sea. My favourites were always stories of a boy on his own, Bucktooth, the Boy Who Lived in a Barrel for example. This character led a nomadic life trundling his home along the road when people or events got difficult and had no-one poking their nose into his affairs or controlling him. When I made him and his barrel his name changed to Derek.

All my hero's at that time were characters who lived a solitary life, giving themselves permission to do as they pleased and finding their own way out of any problems caused.

The cleaners hated my Plasticene because a bit here and there would be trodden on and flattened into the parquet, this they would have to remove by scraping with a knife. Mrs Poole was the chief cleaner and she would complain and say she was going to get my Plasticene taken off me, other toys that fell to the floor she would accuse us of throwing down deliberately, a ridiculous idea, no-one wanted their toys on the floor where, if you were distracted when she came sweeping all before her with a broom meant you had lost them. You had to ask her to please pick the, to her, inconsequential thing up and she would grumblingly comply. This did not suit his lordship, as Mum would say, so I had to find a way of retrieving lost treasure myself.

The edges of the woolly red blankets were sewn over with a zig-zag of woollen thread, a bite through this and a steady pull would unravel a length sufficient to reach the floor, add a hook made from a staple removed from the middle pages of a comic and a lump of Plasticene to add weight and straighten the length of wool which otherwise would have been too crinkled after its previous job with the blanket and most things could be hooked up in triumph. The negative side was that I could no longer allow myself to ask her to please pick up what could not be secured by the hook method and had to make sure I asked a nurse who was passing. On one occasion I even let something go rather than ask her.

The hospital employed a plumber who would often be called to the ward to fiddle with the taps or radiators; he would arrive unannounced with a fixed half-smile and a slightly embarrassed air. I gave him a nickname early on in my career as boys ward guru. This man it seemed to me had the facial look of a certain animal and his jaw-line, added to his interest in all things aqua, led me to name him Hippopotamus. From that point on when he entered the ward a cry would go up of look, it's Hippopotamus! This was perpetuated throughout all my subsequent admissions being passed on to every new intake of patients, and was somewhat remarkable given that the average stay might only be a couple of weeks per patient. Hilarious to me were the kids who pronounced his name Hittapotomus, and on one visit to what was referred to as my second home, all the current crop of boys were using the aberrant form, when I left order had been restored.

During term-time a really lovely teacher would come to the ward each school day, I wish I could remember her name but it is a detail that's lost, however she was very good at cajoling the less biddable, me included, into getting a little school-work done. Sometimes I would pretend to be asleep and while this was initially a useful tactic she would come and look at me with a smile, I couldn't resist peeping, and boredom setting in I would eventually 'awake' and join in with her plans. Once only I took it all the way and stayed 'asleep' for all of her time with us. When she left I felt the most weird combination of triumph and regret, she was a very pleasant woman and I knew I'd let her down, but on the other hand I'd overcome the boredom and lasted unbeaten until time was up.

As ward 'daddy' in the sense that most of the others knew nothing about hospital wards and I had experience of most things I acted as instigator and director of events. Visiting hour started when the screens holding back the crowd were moved aside to let them pour in, I organised the boys to place their pillows on the bed to make barricades against the charging hoard of parents and friends transformed into murderous intruders and we would fire volley after volley from our imaginary rifles until each of them reached the little boy they were visiting their faces filled with puzzlement or affronted frowns with words of stop that now, or aren't you pleased to see me? Some would join in and try to dodge the bullets or say you got me but these were members of that rare species 'fun adults'.

When bespectacled Mr Parry-Williams, accompanied by his entourage, came into view at the babies ward I would often lead the singing of:

My eyes are dim, I cannot see
I have not brought my specs with me.
I have not brought my specs with me!

He would stand hands on hips and with a big grin on his face until we had finished and then start the ward round, here was one adult in our lives who was definitely fun and never took himself too seriously. Once Harry Parry had me taken to a small room where he fitted me up to an electro-cardiograph machine and gave me the information that my heart was being tested, I'd had to wait for him in the room and for the equipment, but was given a book to read, this was an old Mickey Mouse

Annual and the point of one of the graphic stories I never forgot, this involved Mickey and his nephews and a misunderstanding of the word ambush as ham-bush. This both amused me and illustrated for me how easy it was for one letter to change a straightforward instruction into a cause of chaos. The E C G went off very smoothly and was repeated several times, not for the last time in my life I was mortified by Mum's reaction after I told her about it, this should have taught me a lesson but didn't. She asked to see Harry Parry-Williams and started to whimper and ask what was wrong with my heart, he quickly informed her that the reason I had been chosen for what was his first experiment with the new equipment was that my heart was strong and the result gave him a baseline of what a normal, healthy heart should produce. He raised one eyebrow and gave me a look which from where I am now I recognise as empathy for my obvious chagrin, but then thought of as blaming me for telling her.

A standing joke between Harry Parry and me concerned food, if I were for any reason in one of the other three hospitals in the city he would ask which hospital had the most edible food and I would answer Gulson, upon this honest answer he would grin and look at the other members of his group, both eyebrows raised and him leaning back in astonishment. He knew that eating was not an activity I favoured wherever I happened to be, and rightly assumed that Gulson was merely for me the best of a bad lot.

We were fed meat and two veg most days and the hospital was where I perfected the technique later used at Corley Open Air School of eating a little of the leanest part of the meat mixed with a little of the cabbage and a lot of the mashed potatoes, this process would leave most of the horrible, fatty, gristly meat with sections of enormous disgustingly chewy blood-vessels and nearly all of the water oozing, overcooked and smelly cabbage and a little mashed potato. A little of the cabbage and meat would be left on the plate and the rest compacted down and given a covering of mash. Thus when the used dishes were collected I would be told well-done you can leave those bits. On days when the uneatable such as soused herrings could not be dealt with so easily I would simply refuse to eat. Sister Shannon would be called, and this happened with others who refused not just me, she would offer you an ice-cream if you drank a glass of milk first. She was never refused, but neither was she taken advantage of as this would not have been tolerated by the other boys and anyway very few ever refused to eat. I only resorted to leaving everything on the plate when the meal was of something totally revolting, usually I could fake it and no-one be any the wiser. When so many adults have power over you, and administer so much that you would rather they didn't, every time you did things your own way or navigated around a rule was a triumph.

Breakfast on the ward was another mine-field because of the way it was dished up and served. Before it was time for the lights to go up on a new day, rubber, yes rubber, bowls in bright colours were charged with cereal, perhaps two or three different kinds, and the milk, hot or cold poured over them for the whole ward and by the time it got taken round the hot milk was tepid and the cereal in those bowls covered with skin, both cold milk and hot milk cereal was a soggy mass and if you liked cereal crunchy, good luck to you because you would be certain to taste the savour of disappointment rather than breakfast. I learned to ask for cold milk, corn flakes every time as this was the least inedible choice.

On Sage, and later on other wards in Gulson, my possessions were never purloined, I suppose that's why I was so horrified at Dotheboys Hospital, and in fact the only thing that went missing was my pop, an orange fizzy drink that went by the name of Orangeinit.

Chapter 9

The label had a representation of elves climbing a ladder and pushing oranges into the neck of the bottle, which had the same label with smaller elves pushing smaller oranges in and if you looked very closely you could see that there was a tiny bottle on that label. This intrigued me as I thought of this process going on and on smaller and smaller. My first encounter with infinity! Some of the nurses must have liked Orangeinit as much as I did for one night a glassful was missing from the already depleted bottle. I complained and was told of a poor little boy had been admitted during the night and was thirsty. I thought about this and was surprised that they should have given him a fizzy drink rather than take a measure of squash from another child's store and dilute it, but that's how most adults were, unpredictable and a little slow-witted. When this started to happen regularly I peed in the bottle I'd just finished and left in on the locker, the next morning the bottle had gone, and all that transpired from what I admit to be a miserable trick was that once again I was told how bold I was.

We had regular visits from the hospital chaplain and one of these, or perhaps a sight-seer was a man with a white goatee beard and supreme confidence, who wore a long white, or perhaps grey, floor-length garment tied in the middle with what looked like a dressing gown cord. This man was mostly harmless, not pestering to see if we said our prayers or whatever as one of his predecessors had, however he angered me by confiscating a .303 round of ammunition because he said it might fall onto the parquet and go off and kill someone, this had been given to me by Jim Cooper and if it had been dangerous his parents would not have let him have it in the first place. It had been chromed so it was unlikely that it was live ammunition anyway. But this monk or whatever stole it from me as I saw it, probably because he wanted it for himself! Of course, it is possible that he wished me to study war no more.....

Other regular visitors came from some organisation, possibly the Rotary Club, and dished out pencils of an inferior make, the wood soft enough to push a finger nail right down to the graphite, pencil chewers could be assured of a mouthful of splinters, and exercise books with a blue cover and very few pages on which to write, no more than eight in fact, nothing serious could be done with them therefore, although they were a good source of staples. The same organisation or maybe some other provided a beautiful aquarium of tropical fish, and every now and then a man came to clean off any algal growth from the sides of the tank and clean the gravel floor and one day I had something to tell him that upset him badly.

When the aquarium was first introduced to the ward a nurse was given the task of feeding the fish, the inevitable happened and she moved on to another ward passing on the task to another nurse and during one of my periodic stays at home she too left and somehow the feeding lapsed. Next visit I noticed, of course, that the fish were not being fed and asked why, I was told that they didn't need feeding as they ate the plants and that's what such fish lived on. I protested that they used to be fed but was told 'No, they eat the plants', I knew I was right and that they used to be fed, but she was so sure that I wondered if different fish had been introduced so that this less than onerous task could be dropped. I waited until I was mobile and looked in one of the drawers where the fish-food used to be and there it was but his proved nothing however, luckily for me, and the fish, the piscaphile came to tend them. He shook his head when looking at the tank and this prompted me to ask if the fish lived on the plants, by that time I already knew the answer. There were very few fish in the tank and when one died the rest would rip it to pieces in seconds, and once or twice I'd seen a fish barely or very newly dead devoured completely. On his telling me they did not eat the plants I told him that no-one was feeding them and he said so that's why they disappear all the time, we've re-stocked twice! Furious and red-faced he strode off up the ward shouting for Sister, and after that the fish were once again properly fed.

My best times were spent on the balcony which was a kind of conservatory tacked onto the end of the ward, with the fire escape attached. It could be a little isolating but depending on where I was placed I could talk to the girls, always a bonus. Most times I would be on the balcony by myself, rarely did another boy join me but one time a boy called Stephen and me were in adjacent beds. We were both looking out of the window and I suddenly knew what was going to happen in the road outside and what he would say. A Morris Minor motor car came into view and he said just what I knew he would, 'my Daddy has a car like that', exactly the words I'd expected and exactly the vehicle. This was interesting and was a phenomenon I'd experienced before, but the whole sequence went on and on for a stream of traffic, a bike, two more cars, one black the other grey, and so on until I began to feel that this wasn't right or normal and wrenched myself away from the experience, refusing to let it continue by turning away and thinking of something else. What the cause of this phenomenon was I have strained to think, déjà vu, foreknowledge, or what I learned to think of as an altered state of consciousness. Could it be that my experience of events was lagging behind the actual happening of those events? I do remember that a strange dreaminess or contented feeling had come over me. There was a horse and cart belonging to the railway that every day would come up the hill past the hospital, a white dray horse and a flat-bed cart, on this day the horse and cart were part of the flow of traffic I predicted to Stephen and myself.

The man who drove the horse would often break off bits of splintered wood from the bed of the cart and hurl them like darts at the horse's behind as encouragement to climb the hill, I never liked to see it done but had to admit the efficacious nature of the deed, I still have the picture in my mind with the horse's mane flying and his body straining into the collar as his hooves struck the road more forcefully. It was one of the delights of the day, worth more to me than the sight of any motor vehicle being at heart, as I am today or have always thought myself to be, a peasant deracinated and violently thrust into city life, missing the stability of roots.

I had a fun time creating a work of art when an SHO came and asked me if I had any bruises to display to a bunch of G.P's and others who were to take a tour of the wards where they'd be shown unusual cases. I told him no and he briefly had a look to check and then gave a chuckle and told me to try and have one for the next day. I thought about this, then took my coloured pencils and pencil sharpener, ground off some colours, wet my arm and produced a realistic bruise, deep purple and mauve with a little yellow around the edges. The next day when he asked me if I had a bruise to show my audience I triumphantly bared my arm and they sucked in their breath and the SHO looking puzzled said he hadn't noticed it yesterday, but on examination there was no heat and very little pain, I flinched slightly when he pressed it, a nice touch of realism and you could tell the contusion was a few days old by the yellow around the edges where it was fading. When they left he hung back and said well-done. I never knew if I had fooled him or if he was congratulating me on the artistic merit of my painting and acting.

My time spent at home was as episodic as usual and it surprises me now how my home friendships never wavered pre-school. Ronnie who lived further up the street and Brian who lived next door were my best friends at least until Jim came on the scene and the agonising, familiar to many children in those days, about best, second, and third best friend challenged and perplexed. I remember how many times I had to reiterate the hierarchy at my first school, Corley Open Air, as new friendships and alliances caused me to feel uncomfortably disloyal. Strangely I don't remember a great deal about Ronnie and Brian and our interaction except that we spent a great deal of time together. My strongest memory of Ronnie, apart from the wheat pilfering episode, is when we played a game where we put our fingers through the wire-netting into the duck-pen in his back garden and tried to pull away before the ducks, who were used to being fed crusts could peck us; the ducks were quicker than us and his mother made us stop and sent me home in case I got a bleed.

Brian's family and the Haughtons must have been great friends as there was a small gate in the boundary fence between the two gardens close to the house.

Brian and I shared our toys which were often made of brightly coloured wood and involved springs, for instance a dog on wheels with a spring and round ball for a tail that wagged as it went. We both had humming tops mine being lost when I floated it on the water butt watching it slowly sink several times and on letting it submerge completely missed on diving my hand in to rescue it.

Chapter 10

Other toys went the same way, a yacht that should have floated but sank when I left it floating, being forced to go in for a meal, and various smaller things that were drowned when a piece of wood utilised as a raft suddenly flipped over.

We each had a kazoo, an even more curious instrument than usual as two plastic drums, one each side with two tiny drumsticks attached by springs were built in and the sticks could be flicked with the index fingers of both hands with the kazoo held in the lips and blown thus providing a clicking rhythm section to the buzzing as we spoke the words doo-whacker, doo-whacker, doo. As I write this I see before me the merry faces of our parents and hear their chuckles. We each had a toy with hen and chicks on something resembling a table tennis bat with strings going to a central hole from hen and chickens to a ball hanging underneath that when swung gently in a circular motion caused them to make a pecking motion. Our parents used to put crumbs on the 'bats' and I for one was convinced that the birds were eating them. Later I noticed that pecking and swinging made the crumbs fall off and felt foolish and disappointed.

Angela from further up the street was very pretty but I don't remember anything else about her at that time, David I don't really remember at all from that time, though my mother told me in later years that we were all three friends as toddlers and that the three of us would sometimes be bathed together! Another very early memory comes back to me, sitting in a field on a blanket with adult ladies, including Mum, and other very young children, me wearing a sun hat and one of them wearing a bonnet, Angela and David perhaps? Boys wore sun hats little girls bonnets. My mother used to tell the story of how I refused to acknowledge that I wore a sun hat and insisted that it was my bonnet! Knowing my early love of words it probably sounded more exotic.

Last but definitely not least, Jim who lived a couple of streets away and who I first met at outpatient's clinic. Our mothers too built up a friendship which lasted many years until my parents moved to Cornwall. Jim and I would play in each other's houses although I mostly recall going to Jim's. I also counted his sister Marion among my friends but my memories of them both at that time are not very strong, only that we played together and I enjoyed going to their house. I left Jim to last because our friendship carried on once I went away to Corley as he joined me there a few weeks after my arrival.

I was of course, disappointed to find the grass fairly short on starting there having been promised long grass and complained to all, never afraid to show my disgust at any possibility of duplicity, having been promised several times that I wasn't going to stay in hospital the doctors just wanted to have a look at me, which I could understand anyone wishing to do, Derek being the most fascinating child in the world, only to find myself admitted. Often too, being told that a visit to the clinic was not going to lead to blood tests, only to be stuck with a needle.

I had enemies of course, Fred a boy from up the street who stole my toys and had the unfortunate habit of defecating without bothering to seek the necessary plumbing, wriggling his backside to deposit his turd through the leg of his shorts or delving to bring it out between two fingers. He was not in fact an enemy, more of a horrifying but fascinating example not to be followed.

The twins were genuine enemies who pretended to friendship and presented real danger to me. Being a couple of years older and a lot more unscrupulous they used me for fun, encouraging me to follow them up a sloping plank on to the first floor of a building site from which I was rescued by a neighbour and on another occasion tempting me out from the bedroom onto the tiny flat roof over the bay-window telling me to jump and that it wouldn't hurt. My mother saw them looking up and overhearing them calling me to jump raced upstairs just in time to snatch me back from the edge.

Another memory of the twins puzzled me for years as it seemed so unlikely. They were in the street, sniggering and whirling something round on the end of a piece of string. They swung it at me and let it drop to the pavement. It was a white rat with red spots and I couldn't understand why it didn't protest at being swung about. For many years it worried me as no white rat has red spots but that is what I'd seen, I suppose my mind was too stunned at the time for only after years had gone by did I understand that the red spots were blood and that they had violently killed their own pet.

Two things I insisted on, one quietly to myself and the other openly and brooking no contradiction, the former that I was NOT going to die before the age of fourteen, it might be someone else's opinion but it wasn't mine, and the latter that my vocabulary, which I now recognise as idiosyncratic, leaving out the vulgar, was entirely correct.

The wire on a barbed-wire fence was Barbara-wire, no argument, I knew a little girl named Barbara and scratchy wire and she resembled each other. I insisted that milk was pronounced mulk and that the Utility Ware clothing which was all that was available during the after-war Austerity was in fact Futility Ware a little twisted logic can almost be apprehended in that one I think. It may seem strange, I really don't know, but I usually drank milky (mulky) tea and the odd tea-leaf that floated on the surface I persistently referred to as a tea-belief and although others might stir their tea I always stared mine, being under the impression that the circular, hypnotic motion of the tea, once the spoon had moved it, was the origin of the phrase, as once looking at the swirling I found it impossible to look away.

I learned, sooner than was good for me, that although possessed of much wisdom the adult could not be considered a fount of knowledge and often their warnings were best ignored. A haemophilic boy suffers all too many dire warnings! Most admonitions could be merely noted and then discarded, partly as a consequence of the delivery being a flat statement of easily disprovable fact.

Many times I lingered by a road, river or pond just to test the parental postulate that 'If you go by that water you'll drown.' And 'don't go near the road, a car will knock you down and kill you.' if they'd said, could, might or advised taking care, I would not have wasted my time checking the theory, occasionally the courting of potential disaster led to unfortunate consequences listed here as: foolish things for a pre-school haemophiliac to attempt.

If I roll a piece of newspaper into a tiny ball I can sniff it around on a sheet of newspaper, onto and off the face of councillor and big-wig and all over the newsprint. Yes, it works! Oh dear, a sniff too far or rather, too sharp and up the nose with it. Refuses to emerge, never mind - no-one's noticed. Half-an-hour later, a terrible, unstoppable nosebleed and miracle of miracles look, on the scarlet flood a scrap of newsprint. Published already, my son the journalist! Hospital, nose plugged.

Mum: Wait for your brother, Syd'll make a hole through the conker with a skewer. Couldn't wait, sneaked a bottle of eye-drops and tried to make a hole with the dropper. Dropper made of glass, crack, it shatters piercing the right thumb. Hospital, wound checked for slivers of glass, gungy gauze and tight bandage.

Mum and Dad: Never touch those used razor blades you'll cut yourself. Why did he keep them in an old saucer if they were dangerous? Anyway, if he could handle them so could I. Got them! Half a dozen without a scratch, hide them in my pocket. Outside and out of sight, reach in and - cut my finger, bleeding freely! Mum bandages, tells me to leave the grass alone, not to pull at it. Reach carefully into pocket to get the dangerous things out and sling them away - cut finger, Mum bandages 'Don't keep pulling the grass, how many times must I tell you'. Outside, must get rid of them, hand into pocket with extreme caution, careful, careful - cut my thumb, all hope abandoned, ignominious confession, bandage, by now cut fingers bleeding through dressings. Hospital, gungy gauze, required to sleep with hand above head.

Mum: Don't try to climb the chain link fence, you'll fall. Not my idea, hers, but if I take care it should be OK. My intension is to climb over a fence that seems very high but in reality only three feet, shows how young I must have been. Close to the top I'm distracted by the extra challenge of how to swing leg up and over and climb down other side. Foot slips through mesh, lose grip, fall backwards, and hang for a few seconds from left leg which has slipped through tight up to the thigh, fall to the ground, thigh skinned, reddened and sore. Limp away, tell no-one, expect a bleed of some kind but not even a bruise. That's the way it goes, unpredictable, heavy fall nothing, slight knock to the elbow, agony, and hospital.

Come out of hospital, late afternoon, full of beans, ready for action. Mum: Sit on that chair and don't try to get down, I'll get you down in a minute. Leaves room. It's a dining chair, decide to get down anyway, I must be very young as I have to slide my bottom off the front edge and slip down. Back scrapes down front edge of chair. Next morning in pain with a back very badly bruised. Hospital for another few days, only eighteen hours since discharged, so home visit only! It seems likely that there were other incidents before I learned my limitations, but learn I did.

Syd was my hero, Syd the brother who made me laugh, looked after me and could make a toy out of what was available.

Chapter 11

Chickens played a big part in all this, as when the hen house was empty, presumably we were expecting a new intake of recruits, and yet I heard a hen announcing the arrival of an egg, curious, but not without trepidation I looked through the open door into semi-darkness and there perched Syd flapping his arms and clucking, such was the fun he brought me. From folded newspaper and chicken feathers he fashioned ingenious war-bonnets for cowboys and Indians on the dump, more gruesomely chicken feet from a hen that had made the supreme sacrifice, though chicken supreme was unknown to us, would be prepared so that the tendons could be pulled to open and close the claws while chasing the more squeamish of my companions.

I have a strong memory of Syd dragging me in my pushchair behind him over flooded grassland and dragging me across a narrow plank bridge on the axles and with the wheels in the water. I remember the fear. That was my ordeal by water. Around the same time he gave me my ordeal by fire, it was just a few days before November the fifth, so I'd be about to attain the age of either three or four. Children had built a large bonfire at the bottom of a steep slope on part of The Dump and, as usually happened, a rival group of bonfire builders set it alight before time, when we arrived it had burned down to glowing hot embers and scattered flames. We were at the top of the slope but not for long, Syd gave out his version of a rebel yell and launched us down at top speed straight for the flames, I barely had time to wonder what would happen before we were there, he may have intended to go around the fire but through the centre we went, sparks, embers and burning wood flying out on either side. Was I fearful this time? Only slightly, more excited by the exploit, he asked me not to tell Mum, I never did.

In the summer of 1948 or perhaps the previous year, Mum, Dad, Syd and I holidayed at Totnes, Devon. We had been invited to stay with people my parents knew who had left Coventry to move to a farm, the family's name was Brown and they had two children, Sandra and Michael. The farmyard gave me problems as it was cobbled and even as a young boy I worried that I might twist my ankle and develop a bleed, very little damage has been done to my ankles due to my foresight, for which I am glad as a fully functioning ankle replacement has so far proved impossible. This farmyard had one very impressive feature, a horse trough on which floated a little toy rowing boat carved from a solid piece of timber and I pushed it back and forth whenever I got the opportunity, blue skies, a duck pond, love, friendship and no bleeds.

I have a photograph taken on the beach at Paignton during this holiday, a picture of myself wearing Syd's old-fashioned bathing suit which hangs loosely on me and I can see evidence of abnormal knee development, the knees being a little knobblier than one would expect even in a pre-school child. I became separated from my family on that beach and amazed people by my lack of distress, going up to another family and quite happily telling them I was lost and waiting with them until authority turned up and led me back along the beach to be re-united with my family. The mother commented that I didn't seem to care when others would have shed tears. The only other memory of the beach is Syd running along a sort of floating wooden walkway and diving into the sea.

Other memories are harder to pin down to that holiday but I remember an elaborate clockwork object behind a shop window. It incorporated a clock but was much more elaborate, possibly some kind of automaton and was on display rather than for sale. We also visited a zoo; this would be Paignton if it took place during this holiday if not then Dudley Zoo which was closer to home, some other time. Under cover, along one side of a room or corridor was a glass case containing a mouse town with model houses, public buildings, cars, buses and many white mice that ran about in and out of doors and poked their heads out of windows. Now and again they would enter the little vehicles and run along taking cars and vans with them as though they drove, a delightful vision for a child even a child with a mild aversion to mice. Later in the day my anger was stirred when two or three boys stamped on the freely roaming peacocks tails wrenching out feathers and running off with them, I shouted and swore at them. Swearing was something I was pretty good at for one so young, precociously accomplished and confident; more about swearing later.

Two family outings had aspects that puzzled me for years, a visit to Tamworth Castle with family friends Stan and Vi Barrett when, on a landing, a glass case containing stuffed animals came into view, Dad was carrying me and my recollection is that he told me that the two animals arranged in a dreadful fight, realistic blood in evidence, were a lion and a seal. I accepted this at the time but later found it very unlikely that such an event had ever taken place, later again I realised that I had probably misunderstood and he'd said sea-lions fighting. The other incident involved Mum and possibly happened at Trentham Gardens or some other fairly local attraction when she took me paddling down what I believed at the time was a long series of steps with water running down, a uniformed man ordered us out. It must have been a cascade, a decorative feature of a number of stately homes.

No doubt there were other trips and days out that I don't remember but I do recall a coach outing to Skegness and Dad's words when he came in from the pub 'Bob Bolton's getting up a chara trip to Skeggy.' What Mum's reply was I don't recall, but an incident I do, when the 'chara' stopped for a time an enormous sow was standing with forelegs over a bar exposing her belly and teats to my gaze, I asked Dad what they were and he said 'that's his weskit buttons' and quickly led me away. I embarrassed him twice more on the coach but these incidents were told to me long after.

The war and the blitz being so recent and people still resentful of the enemy, what should I start singing over and over but 'I want to go to Germany.' Later, on seeing me eyeing the man in front's head he quietly said to my mother 'If he says anything, I'm getting off the coach. He didn't but I said it 'Why hasn't that man got any hair?' I suppose the answer was 'Shussh'.

It should be plain by now that I was a difficult child, I would fight, bite, scratch and swear if not prostrate when the ambulance came to take me into hospital yet again, I did not want to go and felt betrayed. On one occasion Mum sat me on the dining table to make sure I didn't run away and cleared everything off the table to deprive me of a weapon, unfortunately for all concerned I managed to conceal the tin-opener, the kind with a sharp blade, and stabbed the ambulance man in the back of the hand, I shocked myself as I'd hoped he would pull his hand away, silly, as he could not have expected anything like it, he was very understanding and I subdued enough to be taken out to the ambulance and off to hospital. The old term for a haemophiliac was bleeder, from the moment of the notorious stabbing this ambulance man would say whenever we met 'What are yer? Bleeder!'

On being placated, after yet another bleed, with a ride to hospital in our next-door-neighbours son's car I reluctantly agreed but on changing my mind begged his mother to rescue me, she offered me sixpence as consolation which elicited the response from this pre-school charmer, 'I don't want your bloody sixpence, I don't want to go to hospital'.

Paediatric clinics could also be a strain; they always seemed to involve blood tests, which were carried out at the Path Lab. at Coventry and Warwickshire Hospital. I never got used to them although some members of staff assumed I would, I had to force myself to comply and never being a very compliant child a point would be reached where I'd just had enough of others doing what they wanted to me. One day I ran out of the department, out of the hospital, and out of its environs with my mother chasing me and begging me to be careful. It became quite enjoyable keeping a distance between us and I laughed as I ran. A woman coming towards me engaged me in conversation distracting me long enough for my mother to grab me, I hadn't realised she had signalled to the woman to keep me there, the smile vanished off the poor good Samaritan's face when I shouted at her 'You buggering shit-arse.' a choice phrase that I reserved for my worst enemies. Silly sods would say 'Where did he pick up such language, surely not in the home?' hoping of course that I had. Hospital folks and fogies, I picked it up in hospital along with head-lice and ring-worm!

Shortly before my fifth birthday Mum and I spent some weeks at an establishment situated in Gloucestershire at Kingswood, Wotton-under-edge, this being arranged by Harry P-W, though how or why or under whose auspices I am currently trying to find out but believe it was for Mum to get a rest. The house was quite large although of its rooms I remember

only a small dining room, where the children ate, the bedroom we shared and a hallway with a giant rocking-horse and wide stairway. Of the rocking-horse and the stairway two incidents remain vivid to me.

Chapter 12

It is true that I was small and that the rocking-horse may have seemed bigger than it was but the mistake was made of letting me ride it and I urged it higher and higher, faster and faster with Mum rushing back and forth arms outstretched begging me to stop, naturally I had to make the most of it and rode for the hills, giddiup, giddiup yahoooo! I felt I could ride on forever but had to stop eventually after a crowd of mums and staff had gathered and the wild ride became a bore. As I'd understood from the beginning they never gave me another chance.

The only person I recall with clarity, I see in my mind's eye on the wide and impressive staircase holding a white mouse on the back of her hand by the base of its tail. Her name was Barbara, not of Barbara-wire fame, much nicer and I think she was the daughter of whoever was in charge. She holds the mouse towards me and asks if I would like to hold or stroke it but I decline, we were wary of mice in my parent's household and besides I might have dropped it.

Food in the bedrooms was strictly forbidden but Mum sneaked in biscuits and hid them in a bedside cabinet, swearing me to secrecy, thus reinforcing for me once more that rules are there to be broken, all that is necessary is to make arrangements not to be caught in the breaking. The just reward was that the biscuits became soggy, the house being a little damp and perhaps inadequately heated and I couldn't bring myself to eat biscuits that bend, still can't.

The children, all pre-school and mostly younger than me, ate separately from their mothers at a low table around which the detachable top half of high chairs, minus the tray, were arranged, I took one look and affirmed that I was not going to sit in one of those as they were for babies. A wooden three-legged stool was found for me, a novelty I'd seen only in picture books and I was proud to sit on something previously reserved for Jack Horner in his corner. The next day another child snaffled it and I whipped it out from under his backside as he sat and he ended on the floor, it was MINE not HIS, a claim acknowledged as true for the rest of our stay.

A watery venue, at or close to Kingswood, which we visited as a group, had iron railings surrounding a pit at the bottom of which water swirled and poured, there may have been a water-wheel of that I'm not exactly certain. On one of these occasions I shouted with delight as one of the others lost his dummy down into the water where it floated briefly before being dragged under never to re-surface. I was as prejudiced against pacifiers as my mother; it served the child right for allowing the foisting on him of a disgusting facsimile of the nipple. I'd been breast fed up to the point where I could beg for 'just a spot' according to what Mum, when I was older, embarrassingly told people. Did jealousy play a part in my joy at the other child's loss?

Looking through Mum's papers after she died I found a letter sent to her from one of the other mothers thanking her for returning this lady's scarf which had been left behind at Kingswood. The letter was dated 1. 12. 49 and mentions a Mrs Drew who made sure I had fun on my birthday, so does this mean that Barbara was Barbara Drew? I may find out one day. Mum also kept letters from my father in which he asked if I'd had a bonfire and fireworks on the fifth of November, none of my father's letters are dated but I feel we were at Kingswood for over a month, six weeks? At the foot of each letter were many an X, kisses for Derek! Mum and I stayed on longer than first arranged, how that came about I don't know but later Dad accused Mum of selfishness as Aunt Doris was cooking his meals and washing his clothes in Mum's absence, I hope Mum took very little notice as her every move seemed to be criticised by one or another in the family.

My brother remained my big hero but a lesser star was Roy Roger's The King of the Cowboys. Roy showed his feet of clay when Mum sent away for a toy handgun endorsed by him and what arrived was a parody of the illustration that had led to my clamouring and when on a visit to Coventry he and his horse missed me out and visited another haemophiliac at home. This boy, a friend of mine, was puzzled by the visit as he wasn't a fan; I knew that Mr Roger's publicity men had grabbed any haemophiliac the hospital suggested.

Syd also in time proved unreliable as a superior being, as our heroes will; on the other hand his tolerance was remarkable as he pushed me around in my push-chair and entertained me with his wit and ingenuity.

He had a life before I arrived of course but this seems impossible to a small child during his first couple of years. He owned a static steam engine which I was not allowed near but which I have a memory of seeing fired up and the smell of the methylated-spirit and steam is still evoked on remembering the event, in my teens I discovered this steam-engine in a large box containing a mixture of things that hadn't seen the light of day for many years, this box lived under a work-bench in my father's garage under a thick layer of dust and bits and pieces of ancient motor-car, when I finally acquired the courage to clear away the clutter and open the lid I was so in thrall of the injunction not to touch Syd's belongings, that I shut the lid and never opened it again! Also in Dad's garage was a collection of bird's eggs neatly arranged on cotton-wool in a variety of boxes, but this is an early memory of being lifted up by Syd to look at the eggs from a distance. The other very popular hobby that Syd obviously enjoyed in his teens was fretwork which was used to produce decorative items out of thin pieces of wood. A small hole was drilled with a specialist hand-drill and a thin fretting saw blade inserted then clamped into the saw, intricate designs were produced by removing areas of wood to leave, that's right, a fretted design. Syd also spent a great deal of time drawing, I have no recollection of his drawings but do remember that Grandad was impressed and wanted Syd to attend the art college after he left school, I do remember an eagle painted alighting on rocks, this was as far as I recall painted using ordinary house paint on a round piece of wood, the only other example of his skill we were not supposed to talk about; he drew a copy of an old-style five-pound-note and this was hushed up but admired by family and friends. A very good forgery, not terribly difficult because those notes were white with Five Pounds written on them, a promise to pay by the Bank of England and a signature, if he'd had the right paper it would have been indistinguishable from the real thing. Whenever Syd was deeply involved in anything he would hum, not a tune in fact but just a hum, an almost unbroken sound like a hive of bees, an appropriate simile as that is what people sometimes thought they could hear.

Then he was called up for national service and joined the army. I have no recollection of his leaving but was told that I had a couple of seizures at that time ascribed to his going away, he joined REME and my father hoped that he would learn a trade by which he meant something of real value that would stand him in good stead within the motor industry, Coventry's major employer, but Syd chose what Dad considered the easy way out and worked in the stores. As far as Dad was concerned this was not a trade, and he would often ask the rhetorical question 'Why couldn't he learn a trade?' distress that could have been read as disgust evident in his frown. His criticism was uncomfortable to bear although I already knew that my early hero wasn't quite as heroic as I'd once convinced myself.

The letters he wrote to my parents and I often requested that Gran bake him a cake and send it out to Egypt where he served and these requests along with the information that he was on jankers or in the glass-house that week are all I recall from reading them some years back. And every time a message just for me, please stop swearing! Mum the instigator. One Christmas when Syd visited me in hospital, he came in his army uniform and I have a photograph of him leaning next to me as I lie in bed, I'm not sure which hospital, and I am wearing pyjamas not a t-shirt so it probably was Gulson, he visited me at Corley too, and showed me how to colour the pictures in a colouring book more imaginatively with, for instance little indicative additions of colour rather than the solid blocks I had been using.

I started my formal education as a resident at Corley Open Air School, the intention being three years at the school, what was intended for the remainder of my education I don't know but have reason to suppose that no-one had thought that far ahead.

Chapter 13

How disappointed I was when the playing field did not hold head-high vegetation, ideal for cowboys and Indians, as I'd been led to believe, the only incentive reconciling me to the idea of going away to school.

My first recollection is of a corridor with a little girl smiling shyly at me and the headmistress Miss Caborn, saying 'this is------? We call her Frizzy'. She had fair, uncontrollable hair like a shorter version of an afro. I recall nothing more of the day or the child but assume I was shown round, almost certainly that's when I found I'd been conned about the long grass. I made my disgust known to Mum on the monthly visit but they must have cut it was her only comment. I was never homesick, not even in the beginning; I had become inured to being away from home and had much self-confidence in any new situation.

Miss Caborn had lectured the school on my physical vulnerability and advised that I was to be handled as gently as an egg as I could easily break. I was glad I hadn't been there to hear it. Because of my haemophilic state my permanent abode was the sick-bay and for the three years I remained at the school I had the same bed, kept for me when away in hospital. The open air ethos was maintained by windows always being open for the perceived healing power of fresh air though most were not sick as such.

Unexpectedly a visit from Harry Parry with, W.S.Chinn head of education in tow, took place and when they approached me I pointed an imaginary gun and fired. Chinn just looked worried and Harry Parry staggered I cried 'Lie down you bugger, you're dead.' He grabbed at his chest and fell to the floor, rising up a few seconds later with a big grin.

After a couple of weeks I glimpsed my great friend from home arriving, 'Its Jimmy Cooper.' I yelled being so glad to see him, I knew he was due but didn't know when. We played Tarzan of the Apes together, taking turns as Tarzan and the chimpanzee Cheetah. Playing the part of Cheetah was much the worst job as Tarzan got to order you about and your job was to obey and contort your face into what was meant to be chimpanzee-like by sticking the tongue in front of the lower teeth thus extending the jaw and making chimpanzee sounds which were the only sounds possible as speech could only be achieved with difficulty. Cowboys and Indians also filled our hours, and school during the week, of course.

Our circle of friends included another Jimmy, around our age who had two brothers at the school, Billy the eldest and Teddy the youngest the names of other friends I forget, one had some kind of digestive or metabolic problem that involved him eating a number of bananas during the day and another who was quite muscular and solid for a little boy and impervious to pain. I can see him now, reaching into his mouth for a loose tooth and pulling it out, more impressive to me than it might have been because there was no bleeding whereas I, if tempted to try the same trick would have provoked not excessive bleeding but bleeding that would have slowly persisted.

This same boy accidentally barged me when running up to us as we were looking over a farm gate causing me to bang into the gate, I held my elbow and called him idiot, the smile left his face and he stood without protest, tears running down his face, tough of body he was a kindly and sensitive sort. Sure enough I developed an elbow bleed and while recovering this boy brought into sick-bay for me a pile of slightly damp comics and placed them next to my bed. I eagerly took up a few of them and a monstrous looking beetle fell out onto my bed and startled I snarled 'you stupid bugger.' and he turned and walked quickly away. He kept away from me from then on looking at me sadly when we 'met' at various points and I being ashamed at the time never spoke of it but have never forgotten my rejection of his friendship.

As an illustration of the unpredictability of haemophilia, a contrast to the fairly innocuous clash of elbow and gate which led to a bleed happened when I was sitting on the edge of the sand-pit, moving my toes in the sand as I'd found a 'sapphire' twice before, bits of coloured glass from a cheap necklace or ring, and hoped for more when a tennis ball being used in an informal game of cricket struck me forcibly flush on the mouth. My lips were numbed and when asked if I was alright with difficulty I answered yes but was certain that this would lead to a bleed as my lips had been compressed violently against my teeth. I kept checking throughout the rest of the day and fully expected that after eight hours sleep I would awake to lips bruised and badly swollen, when hospital would be certain as the internal bleeding would have continued. Nothing transpired, not one tiny bruise.

Robin McCalman a near neighbour from home was already at Corley, and although not friends he provided a link to my former life. Robin suffered from asthma and severe eczema, the eczema itched and his skin was ridged and criss-crossed with rhinoceros-like lines. He came to sick-bay to take regular painful baths laced with medication. The toilet and bathroom in sick-bay were together in one room and when I went in to use the facilities Robin was in the bath and I looked towards him provoking 'What are you looking at.' in a very distressed and angry voice, which normally I would have thrown back in a harsh retort but tears were running down a face screwed up with pain and I felt a wave of understanding and saying nothing peed, flushed and walked out.

I was told that before I arrived at Corley Robin had tried to commit suicide by eating berries. This may or not be true; all I can say for certain is that in sick-bay a poster warned of the danger of eating berries complete with illustrations of the various kinds. The story was that he had eaten a number of berries thinking them to be deadly nightshade when in fact they were the less poisonous woody nightshade. Was the poster put up after or before the alleged incident? I can't know, but perhaps he saw it and the attempt was a classic cry for help, or perhaps he'd eaten the berries just because they were berries and he thought them safe or was the poster displayed after the event to ensure the right berries were ingested next time? A cruel suggestion but that's just the caring person I've become.

The only friendly act from Robin was when we were taken down to Corley Rocks and he showed me a water-tower in the far distance as we looked out over the city. 'If you run away make for that tower and when you reach it you'll know you're almost home.' I had no thought of running away, I quite liked the place, it was better than any hospital anyway but I never forgot his advice.

Later when I did run away it was out of solidarity rather than home-sickness and then I didn't get far on account of the calliper I was by then obliged to wear. Miss Caborn had left the school, another headmistress taking over only to be replaced quite quickly by a woman known to many school kids as Old Ma Rushby after a spurious resemblance to a comedy character from the movies Old Ma Riley. Miss Rushby was not beloved by children, as you might have guessed, and looked at as a 'tartar' by parents.

After a couple of my comrades had run-away and been brought back by the police Miss Rushby addressed the school and advised that our running away hurt no-one but ourselves being pointless as the police always brought the malefactors back, she then uttered the words that were, naturally, taken as a challenge: I don't care if you all run away! Later a meeting decided that as Old Ma Rushby didn't care if we all ran away we should do it. A mass defection was the outcome and a large number fled.

I was soon overtaken as I struggled down the road and the car carrying Old Ma and others passed me with a wave after slowing down so she could say 'Out for a little walk, Derek we'll pick you up later'. A humiliating experience but as I'd not expected to get anywhere I turned back to deny her the pleasure of forcing me into the car which would have led to unpleasant, potentially haemorhagenic struggling. Those not immediately caught were eventually returned by family only the hold-outs who spent a night or two on the run suffering the usual punishments. Did they learn a lesson, did Old Ma Rushby?

Cabbages and Onions, how the name of the organised games of Cowboys and Indians came to be so bizarrely named is hard to fathom, possibly the rhythm, of course we played cowboys and Indians in small groups all the time, but the organised games were different. Several of the older boys were acknowledged leaders and had acquired from somewhere poles, similar to broom handles but in my recollection somewhat stouter and longer, these were known as totem poles but more accurate, given one of their uses, better called coup-sticks. The beginning of a game of cowboys and Indians would be announced by the owners of the poles banging the blunt end on the ground and chanting 'Who wants a game of cabbages and onions.' this was the signal for the followers of each to gather round their 'chief', quite what the rules were or indeed if rules existed I never knew but at some point the game changed to everyone trying to catch a girl, most of whom had gone into hiding before the change of emphasis. Only those innocent of what was about to happen or those who knew and quite liked it remained. The 'totem poles' were decorated by the odd large feather but principally hair ribbons and locks of girls' hair. When caught the girl was pinned down and symbolically scalped by being forced to give up a hair ribbon or in the case of a girl not having the required ribbon to surrender a lock of her hair, these trophies would be affixed to the pole and the status of the chief and his gang of ruffians judged according to the amount of trophies collected.

The other end of the pole was sharpened and competition as to which chief could throw what now became a spear was intense. The fun came to an abrupt end when a boy was hit in the head during spear throwing.

Chapter 14

Miss Caborn confiscated the poles and in front of everyone threw them into what we called the swamp which was a very boggy area just over the fence from the playing-field where she knew no-one would have the temerity to try to reclaim them. Did this incident precipitate her leaving and Old Ma Rushby's eventual appointment, I suspect it did.

Common sorrel Rumex acetosa grew close to the ground on the playing field. This, kept short by mowing its arrow shaped leaves close to the ground, was known to us as vinegar leaves, although my mother who originated in Leicestershire knew them as sour grasses. These we would eat following in the foot-steps, I have subsequently read, of old-time farm labourers who would chew them to stem their thirst. I have no recollection of ever being able to squat, so my picking and eating vinegar leaves was sporadic but I remember a craze that swept up a great many of my schoolmates on a couple of beautiful sunny days, squatting and shuffling forward, grazing across the field fully concentrated on the search and cramming the leaves in mouths green with juice, the countryside echoing with cries of triumph at the discovery of yet another patch.

Such carefree joy always seems to generate a downside and vinegar leaf eating, led to aching stomachs and, if you're already feeling queasy I apologise, green stools which the first producers of such called on all to witness. To be serious about all this, the oxalic acid contained in the leaves may well have been harmful given the amount devoured but given the quantities of alcohol and nicotine that many would consume in adulthood, the few days occupied by the Great Vinegar Leaf Rush probably were and remain insignificant.

The hair-ribbon grabbing exploits of cabbages and onions combined with the strange phenomenon of a dish of soap-flakes always kept next to the sink in the sick-bay bathroom gave me, a child with the ability to make original connections, the idea of setting up a laundry for girls hair-ribbons that quickly developed into the Doll's Clothes and Hair Ribbon Laundry, proprietor and sole operative, Derek. This enterprise did not last long and proved a great deal more time-consuming and tricky than I had anticipated, washing being easy, drying problematic involving radiators and being made to remove the drying washing and rearrange again once authority behaved in the way I have always preferred and cleared off. The experience would not have been repeated, it had become a bore and a burden but on restoring the washing to the little girls queuing outside one of the open sick-bay windows it became obvious that the decision to quit had been taken out of my hands.

One of them, a thin little soul with straggly hair and spectacles with a patch of sticky tape obscuring one lens, had given me to wash a strange hand-made garment of green hessian like material. This she got back a slightly paler shade of green. Imagine all the colours that could be changed by a strong green dye, and of a chatter of little girls anticipating clean ribbons and dolls dresses and how happiness was turned to dismay. 'This isn't mine! My dolly has a pink dress.' 'No! My ribbon is white'. And an, irritated beyond all patience, little boy saying 'Just take them; you didn't have to pay, did you? You're just ungrateful, and you (pointing at glasses-girl) it's your fault, you shouldn't have given me that thing to wash'. Now imagine a line of little girls, heads cocked to one side and fists on hips, threatening and complaining, one or two choosing to wag fingers for emphasis and Derek pushing the rest of the perfectly clean and dry washing out of the window and closing it, then stalking off, with his patent severe frown, muttering, 'Only doing them a favour, and that bloody green thing'.

The location of the school, on higher ground out of and above the city, meant that the air was eminently breathable and thought to be very good for those with asthma, a lot healthier for all than the cramped and polluted city below. The air and the nourishing, though incredibly plain, food were expected to, and mostly did, improve the general health of the children sent there.

Next to the gate was a sign which read Corley Open Air School for Delicate Children, physically true no doubt but false in other ways which will become apparent. The main building contained all the things associated with a residential school, the dormitories at opposite ends, at an angle so that the main buildings resembled a box minus lid and with relaxed sides. Constructed of wood on brick pillars the whole impression was one of rusticity. The girl's dormitory as one approached the front entrance was on the left and the boy's on the right, although the angle made things difficult boys and girls could see each other if they stood up on the beds and jumped up and down, and this in fact happened when a pact was made, between genders, to remove their pyjamas and jump up and down naked. I was not involved, fortunately as I would have found the proceeding more frustrating than illuminating! The dormitories had only three complete walls, the fourth being about three feet high, this being the front wall and beyond it a covered walkway with steps, halfway along, to the ground. Thus the sleeping pupils had a full-on experience of the open air. A sudden fall of snow often led to snow on the beds just under the shortened wall and those who were given cough medicine in a glass with a teaspoon could pull out the spoon in the morning and display a cough medicine lollipop. It's true that a canvas screen could be lowered during a snow-storm as extra protection but I never saw this done. When the snow was really heavy and had drifted up to the level of the walkway the hardier souls would run out and jump naked into the drift and then scamper to the showers.

Behind the main range of buildings was another set consisting of staff accommodation, the mattress store, and an isolation area for those who had caught childhood diseases or something else that required isolation. I learned from a correspondent found on the internet that Robin slept in the isolation hut, this was news to me but given the disfiguring nature of his eczema not surprising. I sampled the delights of the isolation hut myself when I and another lad, whose name I don't recall contracted mumps.

After a few days we were sent to Whitley Hospital and shared a two bed cubicle which was devoid of any other thing but us and the two beds and associated lockers. Our 'cell' was at the end of the row of similar cubicles and as it was a ground floor ward, visitors were permitted to stand outside and yelled conversations took place through the closed windows. The row of cells had large glass panels in the wall separating each that made it possible to see right through to the end of the ward, which might have been entertaining, but wasn't. In fact entertainment was nil, and although toys and books could be brought in, they had to be burnt when the patient left. Mum said she would bring in various toys including my teddy bear, known as little Ted. I yelled through the glass 'No, I don't want him burnt!' I didn't want any of my things burned so insisted that they not be sent in. My fellow prisoner agreed. Comics were different and once read were always destined to be disposed of so these we eagerly awaited and just as quickly exhausted. What could two boys, incarcerated without toys and books do?

Here's what, pull the wool off the ubiquitous hairy red blankets and make as large a ball as possible, hanging them from the bed-springs to prevent confiscation on beds being made, and putting them under the pillow when the room was cleaned. We tried to make pets of the strangely numerous money-spiders, inviting them to enter the woolly maze and hoping they would stay, they never did, however often we tried to inveigle them into tenancy but given the materials at our disposal it isn't surprising that we lived with the hope that success would finally appear. We also had a great deal of fun, and this too was my idea, making the nurses come all the way to our cell and ask what we wanted then go back grumbling. We would work through the alphabet finding words that rhymed with nurse and shout the word urgently but indistinctly by sounding the first letter more quietly than the rest of the word e.g. cURSEs or wORSt, when asked why we were calling we were playing a game and shouting curses or this is the worst food yet.

The best time we had was when the cleaners, who had been polishing the floor by means of sloppy polish applied with a bit of stick dunked in a tin and with a flick of the wrist slapped onto the floor, left a large tin unguarded. What a gift! We slopped and slapped until the tin was almost empty and the whole of the floor awash with stuff that looked just like the mashed swede they tried to persuade me to eat. The smell was abominably strong but that and the disapprobation our efforts provoked was nothing compared to our delight at having something so joyously anarchic to do. I always found opportunity in situations others found boring, even sitting for hours in front of meals that I'd been told I would sit in front of until I ate. My mind would be away and playing and plotting revenge, but weeks in that place bored even me.

The silly bit was that somehow or other the kid caught chicken pox and my parents were told that I had to stay with him to see if I could catch it although immune from having the malady some time before. Perhaps the truth was that they wanted both of us back together at Corley free from any disease, or didn't want to deprive him of a playmate.

The school nurses during my time were Ball and Lowe. Nurse Ball treated all the little ones like younger brothers or her own children and would sometimes initiate a tickling session or put her arm around a child and give a hug. Just before one Christmas she was full of her plans to decorate sickbay like the court of King Neptune with simulated seaweed hanging from the ceiling and other delights, this never happened and I assume she was refused permission, but her description and intent delight me even now, and nothing she did was ever wrong in my eyes. While both were wonderful people nurse Lowe was especially good to me, seeming always to understand.

Chapter 15

For many years until it was thrown out by my parents, I kept a birthday card nurse Lowe gave me on my sixth or seventh birthday. It had a picture of a boy leaving home, going out through the gate with a stick over his shoulder on the end of which hung a bundle, she had written Derek on the card and an arrow pointing to the boy, inside she had written: To Derek, my little wildwood flower, growing wilder by the hour.

She awoke me one night and took me through to her quarters where her cat was giving birth, the kittens seemed to be emerging from under the cat's body rather than from inside such was my innocence and although the thrill of being woken and taken to see the event gave me pleasure, I had no clue as to why the treat had been given. When I told my mum about it she said nothing but put on a downcast face and I knew she was finding it hard to understand the why of it. The birthing of these kittens gave me problems in later years, as whenever sex education was mentioned she would grumpily say 'there's no need in his case, he knows all about it already, the nurse showed him kittens being born'.

I loved both nurses and what is remarkable since my trust was hard to win, trusted them, Miss Caborn too. What a splendid head she was, only using her authority when strictly necessary and banning corporal punishment, invariably kind and understanding even when provoked by boys absconding, she seemed to understand. Incidentally I don't recall girls running away though they may have done during the Rushby breakout. Miss Caborn used to give me the odd bourbon biscuit, her favourite, and gave me a papier-mâché Father Christmas too. I only once yelled at her and that was when she entered the bathroom when I was using the facilities, a thing I'd been taught was the height of indecent intrusion.

For a time we had a young French girl working at the school I'm not sure of her status but she may have been au pair. She was a lovely, sweet young woman who adorned herself with a delicious perfume the memory of which charmed me for many years, catching it on the breeze when out in a crowded street and trying to find the source of such an evocative and beautiful scent. She possessed a perfect aquiline nose perhaps a little too large but which suited her beautiful face, and was incredibly kind. She arranged my pillows telling me that this was the French way. Thus when I was confined to bed recovering from a bleed, the pillows supported me as would an armchair. Alas, I don't recall her name only her all-round loveliness.

The cooks and maids I do not recall, or the name of the handyman cum cat-assassin. There were feral cats around the school and one of them, a skinny looking dirty- white queen, had many kittens over the time of my Corley days, mostly under the raised floor of the building. The handyman would crawl under and collar them, drop them in a sack and take them away. One day I caught him throwing the kittens into one of those sewage treatment contraptions with an arm that moves over the circular bed continually spraying water. How I hated him and how certain he was of the fact when I screamed full pelt: You stinking, bloody bastard, you buggering shit-arse. He gave a shuddering lurch and ran back to school. Nothing was said to me but from then on the kittens would be collected by the RSPCA and taken away in a van. I watched once as the inspector crawled under the end of the building and the cat carried her kittens out of the opposite end one by one and got them all to safety, snatching the last one just as he reached for it. This little boy quietly celebrated.

My teacher I remember with pleasure, although her name has long been lost to me. When first I entered the school room I sat under the desk and refused to do anything, she left me there but later brought out the Plasticene, this being one of my favourite things I could not resist and fashioned a canoe with a native American who was pulling along behind the canoe a small raft with furs for trading. This I had seen in an illustration in a comic and copied it from memory, I saw she was impressed. Disney's Alice in Wonderland (1951) was very popular, needless to say I never saw it as the world outside the school didn't reach me, but she had drawn on large sheets of card, kings and queens as playing cards and her skill in producing these impressed me reciprocally.

There was a great deal that was craft related, and a carousel constructed of card by teacher, and coloured by us and horses made of acorns and matchsticks. Nature study played a big part in our lives and the acorns had been collected on one of the walks in the local woods where we also found puffballs to squeeze, filling the air with spores, and a stinkhorn to be nauseated by.

Although already recognising many words from being read to over and over by Mum, I learned to read from a book called Farmer Dan, and the second book in the series Farmer Dan Takes his Farm to Updown. This upheaval in Dan and his animals' lives was accomplished by train and even now one of the many illustrations is fresh in my mind, the horse looking out over the side of the truck. I left Farmer Dan when we started the Beacon reading books, which were full of fairy tales and stories, such as The Old Woman who lived in a Vinegar Bottle, Henny Penny, Rip Van Winkle and the like.

We also created covers for our work books out of card upon which we had painted a loose paste of powder paint, water and flour. We chose our own colours and mine was a violent scarlet. We then cut a toothed edge on thick card and this we used to scrape over the covers to produce a design. One of the books was a diary and I remember the recording of an exciting incident. It was almost November the 5th and of course it was forbidden us to have fireworks in our possession. A boy had a box of Bengal Matches smuggled in and showed one or two of us the delights of these miniature hand-held fireworks. Unfortunately, the next time he lit one authority came along and he shoved it in his pocket where it continued to burn. Bad for him but good for my diary, I drew in coloured pencil, him with jeans ablaze and added the line: Basil Harris burned a hole in his trousers with a Bengal match. This was a nice turn of phrase for a six year old. The diary and other books I kept for many years until they, like so much other memorabilia were thrown out by my parents.

I must have been quite good at simple arithmetic as I was given the task of helping a little girl with her sums. I tried my best but she proved impervious to all my explanations and cajoling, predictably I took this badly and was relieved of my duty when I exasperatedly chalked on her back 1+1 =2.

Singing and the chanting of poetry was also to my liking, and although I don't remember the words one of the rhymes involved turning the handle of teacher's desk pencil sharpener while chanting. I do remember a few words of one of the other rhymes however:

I think mice are rather nice
They run about the house at night
They nibble things they shouldn't touch
And nobody seems to like them much
But, I think mice are rather nice.

That's the total of what I recall, not verbatim but the whole poem I have now found online, entitled Mice it was written by Rose Fyleman and must have impressed me as I've retained the above for sixty years.

One other and cringingly weird memory concerns another teacher, she would stink and look sad and bedraggled, her hair greasy and unwashed every so often. The smell and hang-dog look made me curiously angry and disgusted so one day I made a parcel out of an old box and a piece of string filled it with sand and approached her saying I had a present for her. She took it and it fell to pieces and the dry sand ran out all over her shoes. During this her miserable expression remained and without a word she walked away with the collapsed box in her hands. I immediately regretted the strange punishment I'd inflicted, still feeling angry but with no idea why.

The only other incident I recall from the room in which I was taught is not something I'm proud of, deep snow was on the ground and the calliper causing difficulty. I fell down and while struggling to get up saw and heard one of my class-mates laughing at me, I struggled to get hold of him but he easily evaded me as I floundered, teeth gritted. Break being over I made sure I was one of the first to enter the room, waited for him to come in and threw a chair at his head, I don't know how much damage I did and have no recollection of the consequences. Add to this a day before the calliper when I chased and stabbed a boy in the back with a pencil and know with me how lucky I was not to be placed somewhere more demanding.

I have mentioned my worst hospital experiences and the calliper I was now using, so now seems an appropriate point to reveal how I came to be weighed down by calliper physically and Dotheboys Hospital emotionally and psychologically, the regime being more demanding than even my behaviour warranted.

Chapter 16

For three years Corley was my home and it was there that I had serious knee bleeds requiring in-patient treatment at the horrible Paybody Orthopaedic Hospital. Three times I had the misfortune to be incarcerated there and was alternately badly treated and ignored.

I was around six years old the first time I encountered Paybody and I had only been there roughly half-an-hour when a boy who was in a cot next to my bed somehow got within reach, said 'What's your name, ear'ole?' then shoved a finger up his backside and smeared shit on my blanket. This idiot whose name was Harcourt kept his eyes half-closed and had a horrible grin. I'd never come across such behaviour before or such people and was disgusted and afraid and I was pleased when his question backfired and he was known from then on as ear'ole 'arcourt.

When released from Paybody, at the end of my sentence, it was with a caliper, the right leg I believe, Bizzaro's triumph. I also left with a deep mistrust of all authority figures and a tendency to keep my opinions, once so freely given, to myself. Back at Corley I struggled to cope with the caliper, which went from the top of my thigh to the shoe and had no mechanism to allow the flexing of the leg when sitting so using a dining-chair was a constant fight against the back of my thigh being pinched between caliper and chair, my only relief was to sit right forward on the chair, in itself uncomfortable, and to rest my heel on the floor as sitting normally meant the leg stuck out in front of me and the weight of caliper and leg put pressure on the hip, back and the stomach muscles which soon became unbearable. With the heel resting on the floor, any movement could lead to the sudden pinching and bruising to the back of my thigh. Mrs Morgan, the cleaning lady, noticed my difficulty and she and her husband came to my rescue and provided me with a footstool made by Mr Morgan and covered with a piece of tartan cloth by Mrs Morgan. I kept the stool for years and it featured large in my life long after my time at Corley. By supporting my leg the stool transformed sitting at meals or school work from a miserable tense experience to a comfortable normality for which the Morgans are permanent stars in my personal firmament.....

During my second spell in Paybody, that Dotheboys Hall of a hospital, I was put on traction for what seemed like months, how many I'm not sure. The traction was difficult to bear, as two heavy duty sticking plaster strips each with a tape attached were applied to either side of my calf and then more sticking plaster wound round the leg from knee to ankle, a splint shoved over the leg up to the top of the thigh and the tapes pulled tight around the bottom section and tied to the foot of the bed which was then raised. After a time this became very uncomfortable as the knee was being stretched to get rid of the flexion deformity day and night. The only relief was to push myself up the sloping bed by wriggling but if caught they made me slide back to the tune of much laughter and ridicule. I found it impossible to get off to sleep so had to wait until everything was quiet and push myself up wedging the pillow so that it slowed down the inevitable slip back into tension that sometimes woke me again, usually however I would manage to sleep until morning, re-arranging both pillows and self before my crime could be noticed.

I was not an easy child in any sense and I bitterly regret the time I lost my temper with Mum over a ball of string, this being a necessity at Dotheboys I had asked in a letter for string, unfortunately 'some string' not a ball of string. After the pleasantries had been gone through I asked for the string and Mum pulled out of her pocket a short length of hairy sisal parcel string and a couple of pieces, one only a foot long, of other string. To say I was displeased would be an understatement as once again my temper got the better of me and once again patient, loving Mum bore it, and as usual I felt shame and an amount of fear at my loss of control.

In Paybody a ball of string was essential for status and for the passing of comics to-and-fro. Swapping comics was one of the ways of counteracting the tedious days but asking the nurses to assist was out of the question as they invariably said no and then one had to put up with 'this little boy thinks we have nothing better to do than run round after him' yap. So a system was in place where the comic to be swapped was rolled up and tied to string, sufficient was then unwound to enable the comic to be flung across the ward onto the bed of the other party to the deal. This system worked very well except for the odd occasion when a more than usually idiotic kid decided to cause a breakdown in discipline by taking the comic and letting go of the string or yanking it out of one's hand. Similar problems happened when passing comics from bed-to-bed and a roundabout route would often be the only way to avoid a trouble-maker and or enemy.

The matron of the hospital was a pale-faced creepy cow of a woman, ever ready to lick the arse of the devil himself to ensure her own aggrandisement and be given the ability to pull the wool over the eyes of our parents. Once a day this apparition would appear at the bed foot of each, smile, and ask if you were alright. At the foot of my bed she would say, minus the smile, and how are you? I had quickly learnt the truth that it didn't matter how I was, she would have been pleased to hear a complaint so that nothing could be done about it in as ostentatious a manner as possible. Then the 'this little boy thinks' chorus could be whipped up to deal with me by ridicule and my position rendered even more uncomfortable. On the other hand matron had favourites who would be taken down to her lovely looking quarters in the lodge by the gates, half-timbered and grand and allowed to look through the toy cupboard taking whatever they chose. I leave it up to the reader whether the fact that the toy cupboard was kept in her quarters and not adjacent or indeed in the wards, toys being the material property of children rather than matrons, had any significance.

During this time I officially left COAS without being able to say goodbye to friends or staff and my box of toys was sent to Paybody. Within a couple of weeks anything of value had been stolen during the night, a gold-nibbed fountain pen, a Christmas present from Mr Turrall, an expensive set of watercolour paints and more. Let me be straight about this: the other children were all confined to bed, no names but the staff rifled my toy-box and damn them to hell. Also stolen was a marionette, Muffin the Mule, a popular children's television character, Mum had saved to buy me, how I wish she had waited until I came home. I was off traction and was receiving physiotherapy out of the ward, I left Muffin the Mule on my bed and when I came back he was gone. When Mum came in to see me I told her, and all the boys had their lockers searched to no avail. It is true that one of the other visiting parents may have had my property passed to them before the search but more likely is that the staff stole it as they had my other things. Perhaps Matron's toy cupboard was Muffin's new home.

The application of 'this little boy thinks' with various additions resembled continuously applied torture and at the same time was a tedious indication of the moronic nature of the staff. I know it doesn't sound that bad but it was resorted to on every possible occasion and provoked the bored boys into chanting rhythmically and musically the child's name over and over again until tears of frustration and ineffectual yells of shut-up were dragged out of the victim. They tried this on me but it always failed, although I might be close to giving in I denied them the satisfaction thus making them the victims, and their only weapon was, in my case, soon abandoned.

I was, even at that age learning my own technique of dealing with the world, of being in the world, and knew that the bad times would change to good if I held on long enough.

So what were the sorts of things that drew derision? Virtually anything could and often did start the petty chorus, and you must understand that your 'mistake' could be reviewed and commented on again and again as the fancy took the staff for as long as their pea-brains could retain a memory of the incident. The extraordinary thing to me during my first spell in hell was that one was expected to defecate at a specific time and that one was expected to do this in full view of everyone else. I had not been brought up to crap in full view like an animal or at a time specified by authority, so the first time I needed a bed-pan I asked as I would have done on a proper hospital ward like Sage. In Dotheboys it was quickly made clear that I should only ask when bed-pans were on offer. The thing was brought to me however, but when I asked for the screens to be put around the bed my first experience of the stupidity chorus took place, 'This little boy thinks he's special nurse A., he thinks we should put screens round him when he uses the bed-pan.' Oh, says nurse B he thinks he's different to everybody else does he, this little boy thinks everybody is interested in watching him does he, nurse A? 'Yes, he does he'll soon learn differently.' My terrible misdemeanour was harped on about for a couple of days and, when even these wonderful people realised that it was old hat, could still be dragged out when other 'disorderly conduct' was sparse and disapproving conversation was beginning to lag.

A television was affixed to the wall and one of the rows of beds being under it the occupants could not watch, and in fact only the boys in the middle of the row facing had a good view, not that the thing was on most of the time, only for children's programmes, but I suppose that's fair enough we were after all children. Beds would be moved out so as many of the boys as possible could see; as my bed was near or at the end of the row facing the television watching proved impossible. On first being asked if I could see OK or did I want my bed moved I said yes, it was moved out and sideways by about a foot and I was asked if that had made a difference or did I need it moved further. As the moving had made no difference I said to move it a bit more, please, the nurse did, about another three inches and asked again was that now enough I replied that I still could not see but then understood that I had fallen into a trap and 'This little boy thinks he etc.' started and went the rounds for a couple of days. But whenever they asked me if I wanted my bed pulled out after that I said no thank you! I could mention many other incidents where this technique was used to undermine my confidence but one more will suffice.

Chapter 17

The wall opposite the television consisted of a series of folding glass panelled doors and the columns they were attached to, these were folded open day and night, and during my first spell there I had a bed-cradle placed so that no weight of bed-clothes lay on the legs, the first night I found it difficult to sleep as my lower body was so cold. At Corley where fresh air was also part of cold nights a small blanket was provided that went under the cradle and lay loosely on the legs. Naturally, the next night at Dotheboys I asked for the same kind of blanket. You would have thought from the absolute cacophony of 'this little boy thinks he' tripe that I had asked for an ermine edged cape and a crown of gold and this was never let drop until the bed-cradle was no longer necessary, so my usual ingenuity had to take over. I waited until everyone was asleep, took off the pillow-slip, covered my legs with it and my towel, and that was my life-saver, probably literally if the shivering of the previous night was anything to go by. I would have to waken before the others and redeploy pillow-case and towel as if noticed by the boys they would have told the staff.

Whilst committing my memories to paper I have come to see just how difficult a child I was and what a challenge I presented to a world where children were to be seen and not heard, and unquestioning obedience was the norm throughout a society where professionals of all kinds were treated with great deference and lauded with praise even if their contribution was bloody useless. It could well be that Old Egghead (the Bizzaro Mr) had instructed them to take me down a peg or two, if so it worked to an extent as the lessons I learned ensured that I despised all those with power and those that wielded it more so and learned to keep my views to myself, but the worst achievement was to saddle me with reluctance to tell anyone of my fears, or emotional pain, to ask for assistance or to tell those around me what I wanted. Not until I was in my thirties did this carapace, necessary to my survival fall away completely. From that point on I began to talk and reveal my thoughts, longings and ideas to anyone I could get to listen.

I developed a friendship with only one boy who happened to have the bed next to mine, Hinton by name. We were required to have wash-bags in that place and one day we were whirling them about by the tapes and they became entangled, we both pulled and I fell out of bed and developed an elbow bleed, which was quite severe, from then on my bed was separate from all the rest on the end wall and they put up cot sides so that I couldn't fall out. Of course, there was a prolonged outbreak of 'this little boy falls out of bed and hurts himself so he's had to have cot-sides like a baby.' The boys took this up and chanted at me but by then they knew it was futile so only a few of them bothered and it soon died away altogether. However I was now more or less isolated and as I was never the recipient of a kind word, or smile much less the affectionate ruffle of the hair or arm around the shoulder I had been used to in a real hospital, all I could do was long for the day when I could go home, ignoring staff and boys and doing my best to outlast them.

I had several elbow bleeds while at Dotheboys Hospital, and was always treated as a nuisance whose bleeds were self-inflicted, but this was probably down to their stupidity rather than malice. When I have an elbow bleed it quickly gets painful and nowadays at the first sign I give myself intravenous factor ix, but most of the time nothing was done at that place, on one occasion when I had a bleed into the left elbow, however, they took me to the recovery room and gave me plasma, but not until I was in considerable pain. Afterwards I was sitting in bed holding my left hand in my right and stroking the back of my hand with my left thumb, a technique instinctively adopted which adds another nerve stimulus to interfere with the pain signals and also supports the elbow, when a nurse passing by casually yanked my left arm out of bed causing a blast of pain and told me to stop playing with my John Willie. These words are verbatim, the shock and pain meant I never forgot them.

The next elbow bleed encouraged the vainglorious Bizzaro to try another experiment on me which at the time I didn't understand to be an experiment, only later when I read in the literature that bleeding into a joint would stop automatically when the pressure inside the joint became the same as the pressure in the ruptured blood vessel did I realise that Old Egghead had decided to see what would happen if you compressed the elbow so that room for swelling was reduced, would that diminish the duration of the bleed? Why do I think he experimented, read on?

When I first complained of pain in the elbow, Sister was sent for and she looked, I won't say pleased but gratified to an extent, as she said that Mr Bizzaro had ordered I be taken to the plaster-room next time I had an elbow bleed. Once there a heavy plaster cast was applied to my arm and I was taken back to the ward, the pain got much worse and I could not stop myself from crying and moaning. 'This selfish little boy thinks it's a good idea to disturb the rest of the patients.' and I was moved to a room at the other end of the ward next to the bathroom where I stayed in agony, not relieved by the useless codeine tablet I was given, for at least twenty-four hours. I could not sleep but hallucinated and (I say hallucinated but am not convinced that the manifestation didn't happen even now) by concentrating, moved my cowboy book from the shelf where they had placed it almost into my grasp when I lost faith and it rushed back to the shelf. No elbow bleed has ever been more painful as the elbow carried on swelling but was squeezed by the plaster cast, if I could have done so I would have cut the arm off or killed myself, probably the same thing, but just had to hang on until it was over. Resting the elbow on the bed during a bleed was painful; imagine the agony a plaster cast caused. I have never forgotten the brutal treatment this experiment amounted to. However there are other brutalities remembered with sorrow and in one case with anger even now.

Nurse Bloxcopf was a bitch, I often think that after the war when army nurses were no longer needed they were sold off as Army Surplus, this is the woman I chiefly associate with the practice. She was vicious and mean-spirited and physically assaulted me, and on one occasion was found out when Mum noticed on visiting that as I tried to lie back in bed, after sitting until it became uncomfortable, that I moved very gingerly and she asked what the matter was. I hated to be caught with a problem so answered 'nothing', she replied that she could tell there was and lifted up my t-shirt to discover bruising in the form of the fingers and knuckles of a hand. She asked who was responsible and reluctantly I told her the truth. Bloxkopf and another nurse had come to make my bed, she told me to move down the bed towards the bottom and because I wasn't as quick as she thought I ought to be struck me a heavy blow in the kidney area of my back. I was worried, I had no idea how haematuria was caused but having suffered it once, perhaps twice before, and I didn't want it again. The next morning I could feel heat and swelling by putting the back of my hand onto the back, and as the day wore on it became more and more uncomfortable to change my position and especially painful to lie on my back. Once Mum discovered the obvious fist mark she went straight to the ward Sister and told her what I had said, did this lead to the dismissal of Bloxkopf? Did it? Well...no it did not!

She didn't deny her uncalled for and stupid deed, perhaps the other nurse had already reported it I don't know, what I do know is that she claimed it was more of a push with the fist and that she had no idea how little force it took to bruise me, her skill as a liar matching her inability to control her aggression. I assume she was chastised in some way, but the thing that caused me distress was that they bought my mother off so cheaply. They made her an offer she could not refuse, and although I understand why she went along with it I feel that more should have been done to protect me, they told her she could come every day and nurse me herself, this happened and some of the boys started calling her nurse Haughton, the situation lasted for a while and then ceased, or perhaps it was the end of my second incarceration, in all honesty I don't recall.

Much worse than the punch in the back that I received was how the Bloxkopf beast treated another little boy.

Chapter 18

The poor chap had to spend months on a frame raised above the bed, flat on his back looking up at the ceiling. When he defecated the stool dropped into a tray placed on the bed under his backside for everyone to watch. How he felt about it I don't know but I found it degrading to catch sight of.

In spite of having to submit to treatment no doubt necessary but which verged on the barbaric he was a cheerful boy and often sang snatches of song as he lay there. You, having shown the wit to read thus far, will be able to imagine the boredom of his position, hands free but nothing to do with them - surely Matron's toy cupboard could have provided something - but his parents, being human and loving, and noticing that nothing was provided for him to play with brought in a drawing pad, pencils, eraser and pencil sharpener. Here was a child, I think his name was Chris, six or seven years old who at last had something to do, still flat on his back he explored what his parents had given him and found the pencil sharpener, now I invite you to empathise, remember the smell of the shavings as you turned the pencil in the sharpener, their smell often of cedar and the look as they magically appeared, crinkled and with an edge of colour, fascinating and beautiful, he turned the pencil and watched and smelt the shavings pile up. The less interesting consequence of the process is the production of powdered graphite, and this poor Chris got on his hands, all over his T-shirt and transferred from his blackened hands to face. Finding him like this what would you do? The human thing would be to laugh and clean his face and hands, change the T-shirt and sharpen his pencils and tell him to ask when he needed them sharpened next. I think you might even try to find him other things to do, you, I'm sure, would show compassion.

Bloxkopf screamed, 'you dirty, naughty boy' ran to him, put one knee up on the bed, leant over him and slapped his face as hard as she could forehand, backhand, forehand, crack, crack, crack! Drawing book, pencils, the whole lot went flying onto the floor and tears, almost silent tears, cascaded down his face wetting his burning and bright red cheeks.

I said nothing, I yelled nothing, Derek Haughton the verbal scourge of kitten drowning handymen and interfering busybody women, kept his mouth shut and never protested or told. But I hated, oh yes hated, disregarded my mother's counselling 'Never say you hate someone, always say you dislike them intensely.' I hated Bloxkopf and told myself that when I grew up I'd find her and cut out the dirty piece of offal she had where a heart should be. Obviously, I never did, but up until my thirties, whenever I felt self-disgust, not killing that poor specimen would come back to me as a further stick to beat myself with. Now I see her as a pathetic ruin of a human being more worthy of pity than hatred.

When Mum, in the guise of nurse Haughton, tended me the Bloxkopf beast would get her into conversation on the bus home, managing to get on the same bus and it isn't difficult to imagine my dismay and feelings of betrayal when Mum eventually defended her. 'She finds things difficult because she has pain herself, she has in-growing toe-nails and her boyfriend is giving her problems.' Well, what mortification, the pain she deserved, but I'm not convinced she had a boyfriend, she probably preferred women. It's my belief that she despised men so took it out on little boys who could not fight back, or it could just be that she was indeed Army Surplus and dealing with, mostly crude, soldiers had soured her.

Every morning the day would start with a 'bottle round', a woman possibly a nursing assistant would wheel a trolley full of urinals down the middle of the ward and her preferred method of delivering these was to throw them onto the beds. This was always distressing for me as a haemophiliac as these urinals were not the disposable kind favoured today but were of heavy glass and a blow on the leg could have produced severe bruising or even a knee bleed. This dodging of the morning missile gave anxiety a good start to the day, and if I'd protested all that would have happened would have been a prolonged recitation of this little boy nonsense.

Everything that could have been done for my discomfort was, and while this next example may read as trivial the hurt felt by a six-year-old was very real.

One of the organisations which often sent gifts to Dotheboys sent a toy goods train for the children to play with, on the face of it a wonderful gift, the scale being quite a bit larger than 0-guage with sliding doors on the closed wagons which on opening had goods inside, bags of something and boxes of something else, more of a model than a toy, the problem was that we were all confined to bed so that playing with the whole thing was impossible. The answer was to give each boy one of the pieces of the train, the engine, naturally for the place, going to the current favourite. As might be expected, my eye was on the guard's van and my imagination was already working overtime on the scenario of Derek living on his own in a guard's van which could be hauled to a new siding every time his surroundings grew tiresome. The person handing out the pieces of train got closer and closer to my bed but just before she reached me she gave another boy the guard's van and when she got to me she said 'You can't have anything because you might cut yourself.' and walked on leaving me to watch the other boys explore something new, something new being a stimulus denied us for the most part. Now I know you are thinking that perhaps the train did have sharp edges and authority was only protecting me but think of these facts. The people who donated this to young children would certainly have made sure it was safe, no boy cut himself on the non-existent sharp edges, if that had happened I would have known, and if the idea was not to humiliate me then I would have been given something else instead as any caring or half-way decent person would have done. By the way the train was taken away to Matron's toy cupboard and never seen again in spite of many requests from many a boy prepared to face the sneering rejection which I was not.

One more incident, and this was a demonstration of cruelty if we take the RSPCA's definition of cruelty to animals and extrapolate to young children, it being said that young taste buds are more sensitive than adult, something you would expect nurses to know. Two nurses came into the ward carrying a large brown jar and a tablespoon informing us that Mr Bizzaro and Mr Penrose had decreed that every child be given a spoonful of medicine from the jar. I, being close to the door was the second recipient, and was given a spoonful of revolting, thick, cream-coloured, burning stuff over which I very nearly vomited. The burning continued for some time after the next boy got his dose of 'medicine', the next boy refused and shouted that it wasn't medicine but sauce and then we had the laughter from the nurses and the laughter from those who had not been dosed. Was it a joke? A misuse of power over a bunch of kids when rationing was still in force and many of us had no idea of horseradish sauce, in my family it never made an appearance, or was it cruelty according to the rules applied to animals, anything done that isn't for the recipients direct benefit is cruelty. This was done to us, did not benefit us, was not meant to benefit us, and was done for the amusement of two uncaring, silly women who should have known better. Cruelty it was, minor cruelty perhaps, but cruelty all the same.

Other less overtly cruel things that sent the spirits plummeting were dentistry and haircuts. The dentist worked his way around the ward through an afternoon, drilling teeth with treadle operated equipment that sent the drill slowly grinding through the tooth of anyone needing a filling, I dreaded being required to submit though I can't really say that I remember having to. The hair-dressers I did get attacked by. A teacher of hair-dressing would turn up with his class of trainees and they would go from boy to boy presumably learning as they went, with their instructor prowling from one to the other. How far into their training these young men were I don't know, what I do know is that it could be painful as the hand clippers they used occasionally jammed in the hair and as they moved back the hand one's head would be jerked backwards and the hair well and truly pulled. When it came to the scissors, in my case, the instructor took over; the first time, not knowing this, I expected to get my ear cut and I to bleed and bleed and the ignoramuses in charge of me not know how to proceed.

The day came when I was released from the torture of traction, what rejoicing, kept inside of course to protect myself, and a little fear of the sticky tape being pulled off.

Chapter 19

I was taken to the plaster room and two nurses unwound the tape that had been wrapped round the leg from ankle to above the knee this was done slowly and painfully with many a laugh from them but not from me, and then the two strips on both sides of the calf were ripped off, these two sadists thought it was tremendously funny and the leg was bright red, throbbing and naked of hair when they were through. I now know that there was no good reason for wrapping sticky tape around the leg and that the strips on each side would have sufficed also that the leg could have been soaked to make it easier to remove the sticking plaster; still people of that type must have their fun before any other consideration. Then a brand-new caliper was fitted.

A photograph has me outside in my bed with the cot-sides and Mum and Gran talking to me, it must have been summer but as I look happy and the sun shade affixed to the head of the bed was not deployed it was not a particularly sunny day. The reason sun made me unhappy was that we had to have all the covers folded down to the bottom of the bed to expose as much of our skin to sunlight as possible, we did not wear pyjamas but a T-shirt, always known incidentally as a sloppy-Joe, and what we boys called bum-flaps but which the staff referred to as modesty shorts which consisted of a one-piece kind of knickers or pants held together by four pairs of tapes, this combined apparel left the whole of the forearms and the legs bare. The sun being strong would lead to the metal of my new caliper becoming very hot and any movement touched this hot metal to the skin with burning pain. If you tried to cover even this one leg with the sheet an uncontrolled burst of 'this little boy' would result and the sheets rolled back down to be tucked more firmly into the bottom of the bed. I had learned my lessons very well and did not complain or ask for anything to be done, but sought my own solution. I would casually drop part of the comic I was reading over the leg and caliper deflecting the worst of the heat, the staff should have realised the problem and could have overcome it quite easily, being so adept at wrapping sticking plaster around legs I'm sure they could have wrapped the part of the caliper that touched my leg in a similar fashion, this would have involved a little competence and empathy but those attributes of a human kind were in short supply. All the time I was outside in the sun the sheet of comic paper covered my leg but all the time too I had to watch for a staff member coming too near and casually remove it, replacing it once the silly sods took their ugliness elsewhere, this was nerve-wracking but better than getting burned. In the aforementioned photograph the comic covered calliper and leg can be seen also that the 'sunshade' is down and not arranged to give me shade on the head, I remember now that it was in fact broken and could not be so arranged, as it was never fixed I assume the extra discomfort and possibility of sunstroke was thought, extraordinarily, to be good for me, character building perhaps.

It must not be supposed that every single minute of every single day was torture, occasionally we would be entertained by a troupe of dancers from a private dance school, they would also sing a little, and though somewhat taunting to those confined to bed this was really quite charming. The police once brought dogs and a show was enacted on the lawn with the dogs put through their paces by their handlers.

On a couple of occasions treats were distributed to all the children, these had been bought in by Mr Penrose the other surgeon, not Old Egghead I don't think it would have occurred to him, grapes were given, even to me, and at Easter a massive chocolate egg was broken up and we all got a piece, even a surprised me, I suppose it proved impossible to manufacture a credible reason for leaving me out, the ingestion of chocolate unlikely to cause a bleed.

I have not mentioned the school work we had, there was a school-room but only those able to walk went anywhere near it, all other lessons were taken in bed. We had a percussion band and one of the boys coming from a circus family we had the loan of a tom-tom drum. I was pleased to be given the tom-tom to play, no-one said why I was chosen but I think I was the best at keeping the rhythm. We had to keep time with a piano and a very strange song the words of which were ducks and drakes are very funny birds repeated ad nauseam. We got better and better at the old percussion until even I looked forward to the day we were due to put on a show for the parents, but on the day, just before the show the drum was taken off me and given to the boy whose parents had secured it, he couldn't keep the rhythm and spoiled the whole thing, I sat holding the castanets I'd been saddled with not caring who noticed my non-participation, in the event no-one did, this was yet another humiliating experience for me and an example of the eternal arse-licking mentality of matron and her cronies, I dare say further donations to the toy cupboard were hoped for.

Apart from beating the system to keep the sun from burning my leg, two other triumphs sustained me as an individual and showed that cowed I may have seemed but in fact my head was held high.

The staff spread blankets on the lawn and we were moved on to them presumably to sun-bathe, we were told that we must not leave the blankets. I saw a blackbird fly in and out of a small tree several times and knew it had a nest and wanted to get closer but we couldn't leave the blankets so I organised a rebellion by squeezing onto one blanket then moving the other closer to the trees and repeating this manoeuvre until eventually we got to where I wanted to be. There had been some dissension from the more cowardly types who reiterated that we mustn't get off the blankets but when I and others pointed out that during such a trek we would not in fact be leaving the blankets at all they complied. Sure enough when the staff came running and yelling their annoyance at our getting off the blankets a chorus of we didn't get off them we moved them shut them up and strangely no voice was raised to say that it was my idea!

I had been further humiliated by the teachers when, after a bleed in the right elbow, they made me write a letter home with my left hand, this was barely legible and when you consider I was still learning to write, was a seriously stupid thing to force on me, this was the letter in which I'd asked for string, it was remarkable that Mum managed to read it and when she died I discovered it in her box of old letters. This cleared up a minor mystery as Elsie Roberts had once remarked that Mum had shown a letter I had written to her and the writing was terrible though Mum had been proud. I'd never claim that my handwriting, or as it was at the time printing, was good but terrible? Well, it was terrible in that letter, practically unreadable! I got my revenge by cheating in the mental arithmetic test, hiding in the sheets one of those exercise books that had weights and measures and times tables printed on the back. I still have the school report, again retrieved from Mum's personal papers, that shows arithmetic fair, mental arithmetic excellent and they didn't wonder about the disparity! At the time of the test I was quietly jubilant having put one over on the whole boiling.

In an attempt at balance I should say that the girls were said to have a much better time than the boys and this has been confirmed for me just recently when I got in touch with someone who had several admissions to Dotheboys, she told me that she was always well treated. The sound of genuine laughter and fun that came through to the boys did indeed cause us to believe that the girls were treated much better than us. My local newspaper carried a mini-series about the place and most of the comments appeared to come from boys who remembered the treats and not the knocks. Only one comment was half-way critical when one old boy said the treatment dished out was harsh but fair, I'd say yes to harsh but fair it was not. It cannot be fair to treat captive little children harshly.

Of all the places I have been obliged or chosen to spend time Dotheboys Hospital is the only one to hold no memories of fun or pleasant times, apart from those organised by outsiders or parents, or any charitable, pleasant people, and make no mistake all establishments, yes even today, where patients or inmates of any kind abide long-term is likely to offer attractive employment to undesirable elements and needs regular, unannounced, impartial scrutiny by an outside agency.

Near Sister's office situated between the boys and girls ward stood a large glass case of stuffed birds, animals and insects which illustrated the nursery rhyme Who Killed Cock Robin, this was a suitably macabre decoration for a place wherein so many had been pinned in place and stuffed to the eyeballs with bull-shit.

In between the two incarcerations at Dotheboys I returned to Corley, my days not quite so carefree as the calliper was difficult to live with in many ways, slowing me down making even short journeys fraught with the possibility of catching my calliper stiffened leg on an obstacle precipitating a fall.

In the dead of winter Reverend Goslin would come to the school on Sundays and deliver a short service, during the rest of the year we would be lined up and given a penny each to put in the collection plate, then marched crocodile fashion down the lane to Corley Church, a lovely old building smelling of polish and damp. Rev. Goslin fascinated me because when sermonising he stuck his neck out suddenly for emphasis and owing to mishearing his name as gosling my imagination was stirred into wondering if he had chosen his career on noticing in a mirror how goose-like he appeared. He would ask if anyone's birthday had occurred since the previous week and if the reply was in the affirmative the child would be allowed to ring the church bell, with assistance, once for every year of age. I never did, was I in hospital for my birthday, was it forbidden in my case, so much was, or did I voluntarily forgo the pleasure as likely to cause a bleed?

Around Christmas a Magic Show was put on by a conjurer who instructed his audience to watch coloured handkerchiefs move all around the room just under the ceiling from one box to another, one boy refused to be distracted and carried on watching the conjurers hands seeing him quickly transfer the handkerchiefs and shouted out 'he's cheating'. I must have annoyed the man, as many others during my schoolboy career; it takes a trickster to know a trickster.

My father paid five shillings a month for me and I suppose this went towards the little treats we enjoyed.

Chapter 20

One shilling and three pence a week didn't go far when you take away a penny for church, three pence to spend in the shop, the few boiled sweets before bed, and the piece of fruit supplied daily.

There was, at that time, a shop in the village and we would be given our three pence and marched down to spend it once a week, three pence even then did not buy much and I suppose some of the children had extra given them by relatives and could have their choice. The pittance handled by the rest of us could buy a packet of crisps, or better than that a packet of ice cream wafers which could be eked out and eaten one at a time, a method sound in the planning but sadly requiring too much will-power in the execution. There were, presumably, other choices but if so I don't recall them, the only certainty I have is that there were very few. The church and the shop were the only legitimate reason to walk the lane, although sneaking out to Corley Rocks was a constant temptation and one we were always glad to give in to, only being taken there once by the school.

Others often shared sick-bay with me, one boy who showed us horrific holes in his thigh which were healed dog-bites, or so he told us and Lawrie who lay still in bed and seemed very weak but sang quietly 'There'll Be Blue Birds over the White cliffs of Dover' with a sad and wistful expression. I went off to hospital and when I came back he was no longer at the school, I surmised, having seen death before, that he had succumbed to whatever his problem was, I never asked after him because if I didn't know then everything might be all right.

In dormitory or sick-bay laughter was always heard after lights out, as jokes were passed around, mostly filthy, I didn't understand many of them but joined in nevertheless, these were the jokes that the nurses liked me to repeat on Sage, rewarding me with the oft repeated 'Ahh, you're a bold boy'. There follows a sample of the more innocuous ones.

First the parrot jokes, relationships between old ladies and parrots seemed ubiquitous back in the fifties at least as far as the jokes were concerned. An elderly woman with a parrot on her shoulder, presumably a fan of Long John Silver, gets on a bus and notices a sign reading no pets, she thrusts the parrot into her generously proportioned drawers, the parrot making no protest until the bus conductor (such individuals took fares and kept order) cried 'lovely day madam' when Polly screamed 'It may be lovely out there but it's wet and windy down here.'

An elderly lady is late for church, rams on her hat, sticks her parrot on her shoulder, and arrives to sit right at the back. Just then the congregation rise to sing and burst forth with Stand up, Stand up for Jesus to which the enraged parrot yells 'Sit down, sit down for Jesus, the buggers at the back can't see.'

Most fauna got a look in somewhere and the next two jokes concern fowl and a dog respectively. A man carrying a small crate attempts to enter a bus and being jostled drops the crate which bursts open. With many a cackle and feathers flying out pop a young hen and cockerel and flutter off down the street. The young man shouts 'Catch me cock and pullet'.

There are other jokes I recall from that time, concerning rubber balls and liquorice, a little dog called Titswobble, a pub called The Red Cock Inn, and worse, but we've had our sample and the rest must remain locked in memory. There were songs and rhymes too.

There is a cabbage dump
Not far away
Where we have bread and scrat
Three times a day,
Egg and bacon we don't see
Jelly fishes in our tea
That's why we're gradually
Fading away.
The nurses they are barmy
The teachers just as bad
Especially Old Ma Rushby
She drives you flippin' mad.

Now to incite a scunner, if the preceding ramblings have not yet done the trick, this rhyme splendid in its vulgarity may!

I'm a little choir boy
I don't swear
Shit, bugger, arsehole
I don't care.

One more:

Tarzan swings, Tarzan falls,
Tarzan breaks his cast-iron balls.

Such innocuous jokes and rhymes whiled away the hours and enlivened the tedium endured by us entirely innocent little children, besides it took the place of outright disobedience and rebellion, a scurrilous safety valve.

Two older girls once had the beds next to mine and I was intrigued to hear their conversation, obviously concerning a secret, one said 'I don't like those other things you have to shove 'em right up you.' alas I heard no more as they noticed and told me off for listening.

Potentially dangerous things happened to me in sick-bay, I came back to my bed to find a yellow 'Smartie', carefully placed right in the middle, I thought Jim had left it there for me, put it in my mouth and bit into it, whatever it was, it was no sweet it was bitter and medicinal. I spat it out and went to the bathroom to brush my teeth and rinse my mouth. I said nothing, hoping that whoever had put it there would give themselves away by unsubtly asking if I had found a sweet, no-one did and it appears that the thing was put there with malicious intent. One day a boy a couple of years older than me came into the room and suggested a new game, I had to get into bed cover up my head and he had to prevent me getting out. So we played, he got on the bed once I was hidden under the covers and swarmed over me holding me down until I found it hard to breath and started to yell at him, he relented and let me up telling me he was sorry and would go a bit easier next time, so I complied and the same thing happened only now I had to struggle harder to get him to let me out, he assured me it was a good game and said to do it one more time, I swore at him and he left. I'm sure his intention was to cause me deep alarm or possibly more.

The other danger came upon me from within; I'd had a knee bleed and was confined to bed with a bed-cradle to keep the weight of bedclothes off my leg. I needed to use the urinal and on doing so felt like I was passing lumps, these turned out to be blood-clots and the urine looked like port wine, I knew I was bleeding from the kidneys and hid the urinal under the covers for hours then had to give in and let the nurse see, hospital followed. I knew what was happening so perhaps I'd already had a session of haematuria before.

The feral cats tended to be a nuisance more than anything, coming through the windows in the night and lying on my feet but one night I woke to feel one of them walking up the bed towards me and when I lifted my head it snarled and rushed at my face, I quickly pulled the covers over my head and felt its teeth and claws scratching and biting the bedclothes before it jumped to the floor. Now this was a particularly ungrateful act, as my main meal invariably ended up outside in the flower-bed underneath the sliding window next to my bed and the feral cats made short work of the meat. I didn't eat much if I could help it as I saw no value in wasting time and energy on eating stuff I didn't like, even now I rarely feel hungry and if busy I am likely to miss out a meal altogether.

Danger called again when Jim came into sick-bay and asked me to knock him out, if I could. I didn't want to hit him after all he was my best friend but he wanted to find out what it would be like and begged me to try. The beds were close together and Jim sat on one and I sat on another facing him. There followed another of those strange incidents in my life where I knew instinctively what to do, I didn't swing a punch as when we played at fighting but hit him with a classic right hook, twisting my wrist just before contact, concentrating everything that was in me on one explosive instant. Jim flopped back on the bed, eyes closed but moving backward and forward under the lids. After a minute or so he opened his eyes and said 'You did it.' stood up and walked groggily about asking me what he looked like. I should probably have been rewarded by bleeding into the tissues of the hand or an elbow bleed but this did not happen. Many years later, when I took my wife to meet him and his parents he recounted the story and said he hadn't thought I would be able to do it; this convinced me at last that his reaction had not been faked.

Jim and a mate once ran away and reached his house, crept into the back garden and hid in the greenhouse until given away by the cat which was sniffing round the door and mewing, my mother happened to be visiting and became suspicious, once she looked in the greenhouse the two were collared and sent back to Corley. Punishment wise they got the full treatment, being required to do numerous chores as penance, the most onerous of which was scrubbing all the tables in the dining room These were long trestle tables that while clean of food and drink debris didn't look as though they had been scrubbed once in their overly-long lifetime. The two also had to spend break time sitting on a chair in separate areas forbidden to speak, the rest of us being forbidden to speak to them. Naturally I found plenty of opportunity to ignore this.

Chapter 21

Not overtly ignoring instructions of course, I endeavoured to take care not to be noticed as punishment heaped on my head would have only been appropriate but I couldn't take the chance on getting them into further difficulties.

Monthly, was it, the visits from parents and family? I believe it may have been, or perhaps fortnightly, at any event in the gap would come parcels from home; Jim's and mine would invariably be the same. Same wrapping paper, same sweets, and almost always a packet of Iced Gems, little biscuits with a swirl of icing on top, only the comics were different so that we could swap. At the time I suspected that these parcels were put together by Jim's mum, known to me as Auntie Gert, I remember being slightly embarrassed that this should be so but grateful too. The discomfort of knowing that my parents had been assisted in their care of me and wondering why that should be accounts, I can only hope, for the fact that I never thanked them……

A very strange boy by the name of Hornet, known to us as Hornet the cornet used to receive a big jar of sweets in his parcel, presumably all his family contributed to it, using their sweet ration. On receiving this he would take large handfuls and throw them up in the air shouting 'scramble' and dozens of boys would oblige. He would keep this up until all of them were gone or the others had got tired of it.

Mealtimes meant a mug of what purported to be tea, its colour resembled water left in a bowl after the washing-up and it had a very curious taste, not unpleasant but nothing like the taste of tea. Into this wondrous beverage Hornet the cornet dipped his bread and butter and smacked his lips as he slopped it into his maw. This performance was always greeted with derision mixed with awe that anyone could like such a mess, I suspect that both of his party tricks were designed to win over the crowd as he never seemed to have any real friends, but if so all he really gained was momentary notoriety.

The happiest memory of sick-bay was when an older girl, who I thought very much a grown-up, read to me. The only stories I remember were amusing ones, a series of stories involving a charlady whose catch phrase was 'No, not if it was ever so!' and a story about a man who, seeing pears for sale outside a greengrocers went in the wrong door and asked the shoe-maker for a pear, confusion reigned over colour, size etc. But the verse she read me was the biggest thrill and Alfred Noyes' The Highwayman, in particular: 'The road was a ribbon of moonlight looping the purple moor.' I could see the scene in front of me as romantic and tragic as if I was there. Her name was, I think, Lorna and to this day I remain grateful for her input.

The kindness, support and education for life I received at Corley contributed greatly to my character and provided the early foundation of my interests today, poetry, and books in general, the natural world both fauna and flora which stimulated my gardening obsession, folklore and music. Some days we had folk dancing and sang, probably Bowdlerised, folk songs such as Henry My Son and others. Every morning we had to make our beds with hospital corners and general neatness, having seen beds made in hospital on very many occasions this was not the most difficult trick to learn and satisfying to see the end result as good as that achieved by any adult. For the bed-wetters among us there wasn't any punishment but responsibility was engendered by making them drag the mattress to the mattress store and bring back a new one. This usually worked a miracle, the humiliation being a strong deterrent; fortunately I never had to suffer this. Other hardships for some were the open-air aspect, overcoats were not worn unless the temperature was really low, and we would be told to run and jump up and down and we would soon get warm. A stoke -hole at the end of the classrooms fired the heating for the school and the handyman would be down there stoking whilst up above hovered a number of girls huddling together around the escaping heat, these were, if noticed, shooed away and the same thing happened to anyone, usually girls, hanging around the radiators indoors, they would be sent outside with the usual advice about getting active. During the summer months we boys invariably wore only pants, shorts and sandals while the poor girls were forced to carry on with vest, liberty bodice and gingham dresses, when they must have been uncomfortably warm.

Confiscations were always accompanied by the promise 'When you leave you'll be given it/them back.' In my case this never happened, which may well have been because when my leaving day came around I was incarcerated at Dotheboys, where my box of toys had already been sent!

The first thing taken away was a rounders bat like a small cricket bat. I felt guilty about this as Jim and I had both been given identical bats on the same day and his was taken along with mine. The explanation being that I might get hurt, for me fair enough, but not for Jim, hence my guilt. Gran on coming to see me gave me a miniature penknife, quite sharp but not razor-like by any means with a small blade, I was so proud to be trusted with it after earlier exploits with sharp objects, but it lasted only until noticed by one of the staff. If I'd known that they were allowed to steal something given to me by Gran, they would never have seen it. However I could see the sense in their fear. Two other confiscations puzzled me at the time and seem even more ridiculous looking back. Syd gave me his trilby hat, which in his role as spiv and sharp dresser had been part of the outfit, coming to his senses and now a married man; he presented it to me suitably banged up into a shape ready to wear as a cowboy hat during our favourite game. This was removed without explanation as something I couldn't have, and another hat of sorts, an old style leather flying helmet which another boy gave me and I used in flying games but which also figured as a deep sea diver's helmet was snatched away with the same lack of explanation apart from 'You can't have that'. This reinforced my disgust at the arbitrary nature of the power wielded by authority, the hats being misappropriated post Miss Caborn.

The persecution I faced from those determined that I should eat was sustained, oppressive and ultimately futile. The burden of the chatter that my refusal generated was that I was only seeking attention, this was of course complete nonsense, attention was the last thing I desired. What I ate and when I ate was my business and no-one else's, I very rarely, if ever, felt hungry even when up and about and expending energy being chased in my red Indian guise by hoards of blood-thirsty cowboys. I used to feel that it would be wonderful to have a little door in my abdomen so that I could open it, pour in the plates of horrible tasting muck or good wholesome food as authority insisted, and get on with playing the part of Big Chief Derek. The waste of time that eating was drove me to despair and I took pains to shorten the affair, pinning an old crisp bag inside my shirt and spooning the offensive meat and cabbage into it, and when the bag reached the point where to fill it more was to court disaster I ate as much mashed potato as possible and covered the majority of meat and cabbage with a thin layer of mash, arranging a plate that seemed relatively empty, just a few little bits of meat and cabbage and a desert spoonful of mash left over, very good really for a child notoriously difficult with food. It should be obvious from this that attention was the last thing required to pull off the trick. If my reluctance to eat had been said to be because this was something impossible to force on me against my will, when so much was, I would have to concede that that probably was an element but my main reason was not feeling hungry and not seeing the benefit of eating what I didn't enjoy. Eating for taste was my thing, and one day I passed the staff dining-room at teatime and saw on their table a glass dish with something black standing up in peaks. 'What's that?' A member of staff chuckled and said do you think you would like it, buttered and spread a little on a slice of bread and gave it to me, starting me on a lifelong love of Marmite or yeast extract. If I liked the taste I would eat in spite of not feeling hungry.

Chapter 22

The packed meals, doorstep sandwiches never Marmite although they now knew I liked it, provided by the school would be swapped for the more delicious stuff Mum brought with her when, on my return from Dotheboys she was asked to take me out for walks in a wheelchair as I couldn't get around much, we must have covered all the lanes in the area and the change of scene was very welcome. Those lanes when I go up to Corley these days and drive around them have an almost magical feel for me and I remember how each new vista of field and woodland and the extraordinary holly hedges native to the place, gave me immense pleasure. A word about the air quality, it being the highest point close to the city even now when I park the car in a certain gateway where Mum and I once ate our picnics, with the windows rolled down the pure air is invigorating and engenders a feeling that this is the right world I'm living in overcoming my usual feelings of impermanence and alienation.

Although my world now consisted of Corley and hospitals the world outside managed very nicely without my interference. There was a little matter called The Festival of Britain of which I knew nothing apart from seeing a few stamps, and a change of government which had no consequences observable from school. In the family, time played its usual tricks, Grandad died and my brother came home from National Service and married. When told of Grandad's death, although sorry he'd gone and wishing it wasn't so, I could not cry even later when alone, as I'd been told by Mum when younger that I mustn't cry, common-sense now tells me that this was the probable reason, at the time I thought there was something wrong with me and a few years later I wondered, when I read of sociopaths and psychopaths, if I might be what I'd heard referred to as an unfeeling monster. Missing Syd's marriage was worse.

Worse because authority prevented my going to the wedding, not because I objected to the marriage or Syd's choice of bride, his wife Violet known as Vi was always very kind to me during my younger years. The rigid adherence to the principle of only allowing a minimum home contact through visiting at the school was surely, in cases of family events, mistaken. I believed right until the day of the wedding that my brother and parents would take me away for at least a couple of hours by force; they had in fact, offered to collect me just for the ceremony and bring me straight back but the school refused. On the day I waited for Syd to come and get me and when it became obvious that this was not going to happen, I felt abandoned and very angry and decided to fight the school by sitting out in the field refusing to come in for meals, and meant to stay out of there for good or at least until they used force when I would fight until subdued. Fortunately it didn't come to that as Nurse Lowe came and talked me out of it, walking back into the school with me. It was touch and go however and any comment from other members of staff would have provoked total rebellion.

I have left my chief tormentor until last in the negative aspects of Corley. I refer to the strange girl named Shipperbottom, who herself was the subject of much torment from those who changed the double P to double T. I could never understand why she hung around with me or followed me about, was she friend or fiend, I suspect more of the latter when the spirit moved her. She even followed me into hospital, often within an hour of my admission she would be brought in suffering from a severe asthma attack, blue in the lips and heaving and straining for breath. This was no coincidence and many asthmatics at Corley knew how to bring on an attack, though of course it probably came down to autosuggestion. I was told by one of them shortly after my arrival at school, that if I wanted to bring on an attack the trick was to sip a glass of warm water, jump up and down on the bed, sip more, jump more and soon enough the attack would start. While this information had novelty going for it I found it hard to imagine why anyone should want to cause themselves breathing difficulty.

Shipperbottom followed me around but her interest, though flattering was quite unwanted. Someone sent me a wonderful money-box with a mechanical system that counted pennies as they were dropped through a slot, flagging up the number until one hundred when a trapdoor would open and out would pour the pennies. On coming down the corridor after being outside, unaccompanied for once by my companion, I saw my money-box lying in the corridor in full view, the trap-door broken open and the few pennies gone. I suspected her but couldn't prove it, anyone else would have hidden the thing but this had been left where I would be sure to find it, her usual modus.

One day she suddenly approached and asked me to come and look at the sticklebacks in a tank in one of the classrooms which I knew we were not supposed to enter but as she had already been in there and my curiosity had been aroused by her 'Come and see what someone has done.' I readily went with her. The aquarium stank and had dead fish floating on the surface and dead earthworms rotting on the bottom, the dead fish were the lucky ones as the ones not quite dead had earthworms sticking out of their mouths and in some cases out of their vents. It was a horrible sight and smell and it upset me very much. 'Let's go' said she and we went.

A couple of hours later the new teacher who had set up the tank, Mr Rees, came to me incandescent with anger and asked me what right I thought I had to feed complete worms to the fish, I had no right to be in the room anyway, and he had never met a crueller little boy. I tried to protest but he wouldn't listen telling me I'd been seen, this puzzled me as no-one could have seen me do what I had not done. Not until I'd left Corley did I see the truth which had been staring me in the face and dogging my footsteps for a couple of years. The person who took me into the room had then gone and lied about seeing me do this thing, having already done the deed herself! Now it all made sense.

At my next school Mr Rees was the science teacher and it was clear that he didn't like me. After science one day I lingered by his desk trying to screw up the courage to tell him my theory about the fish and plead my innocence, this was a big deal to me because then he would have known my concerns and might have used them against me in some way. In the end it didn't matter as he curtly said 'on your way, Derek' and I went, never to attempt to talk to him again.

During my early years and the first three of my education I met so many adults, a great many forgotten but others who had a great influence on me and a few whose presence was a recurring theme, the visiting physician being one.

Chapter 23

Dr Gaffney was one of Mr Parry-Williams crew and came to check our health regularly, I remember having to strip and drape myself in a blanket prior to her examining me, she held my scrotum and bade me cough; this seemed a strange procedure but as a quirk of character, could have been worse, so I obliged. She opened a drawer and got something out, I don't remember what, but I was glad it wasn't a tongue depressor as there was a wet patch in the drawer and several droppings accompanying a strong smell of mouse, neither of us mentioned it.

Mum was forever quoting the family G. P. on my early death in my presence and Dr Gaffney told her 'Nonsense we'll both be here to dance at Derek's wedding'. She went on holiday and brought me a book called When I Grow Up; it had descriptions of many jobs and exciting coloured pictures. The only one I recall, and I recall the picture in detail, had the captain of an ocean liner, wearing a big and confident smile, standing next to a large vessel that loomed above him. I never doubted that I would grow up, but most of the careers were impossible for me to imagine for myself, just think of the Master of a ship, having a bleed somewhere out in the Atlantic, or a postman getting a knee-bleed at the beginning of a round or.........well, no need to go on, most jobs seemed unlikely and the one or two available as far as haemophilia was concerned interested me not the slightest, I knew that if I ever had a job to give to someone it wouldn't be a haemophiliac. This set me up for the greatest betrayal of my life, several years in the future when I was almost out of the clutches of Acts Educational.

But for now although out from the clutches of Dotheboys and my first school experience over I was still subject to the whim of educators and medicine men (and women). I have never fully forgiven the ineptitude that saw me sent away for three years then failed to give me the opportunity to say my farewells to loved staff and friends at Corley. I arrived home directly from Dotheboys; caliper encumbered and found nothing was prepared for me. A uniform had been supplied at Corley and obviously after three years I'd outgrown my old clothes so for many months wore the sort of thing you see in movies about hillbillies or share-croppers, a sort of dungarees though theirs were made of denim and mine made by Mum from an old coat of my brother's, this was not as bad as it may seem because at least the garment covered my legs and put a stop to the pitying looks.

Mum did her best in difficult circumstances, the main difficulty being a lack of money, when I returned from Corley austerity measures following the war were still in place nationally and in our place carried on long after every other home gained relief, I saw my mother's struggles as she tried to manage on the money dad provided which had, I imagine, not increased since the war.

Many things others took for granted were treated as exotic or at least unnecessary, biscuits, fruit, and toilet paper. A stack of old newspapers rested in the bath and bits had to be torn off to do the necessary. Compared to my friends I lived an increasingly primitive life and as time went on so the disparity increased as various things fell apart and were not replaced, here's a curious one, we didn't own and presumably never had owned, nut-crackers, well, anyway this didn't usually matter as we only owned nuts at Christmas, but the method of nut cracking was unique as far as I know! The nut would be placed on the tiled hearth, just in front of the fire and the iron, yes the one used for ironing clothes, would be brought down in a controlled fashion to crack the nut without mashing it into the tiles, a skill that had to be learned in the same way youthful chimps learn when using two stones as hammer and anvil, when I see film of this I have to grin at the resemblance to me and my family or vice versa. The 'hammer' was not an archaic flat iron but a broken electric iron which had to be heated up on the hotplate of the electric cooker. Mum would test for the correct heat by moistening her finger at her mouth and touching it to the base of the iron, a good sizzle meant the correct temperature had been reached and as it cooled she would repeat the process until the ironing was done. This was achieved on the dining-table, we didn't run to exotic clutter such as ironing boards.

I dragged the damned calliper for at least another year and when set free found it impossible to walk without holding the leg as rigidly straight as the calliper had held it. Flexing the leg when sitting was not easy and could only be accomplished by gradual relaxation and massage which my father would observe with concern and a degree of, I felt, irritation. Knee bleeds were common during the next few years and often one or the other of my legs would be encased in a full length plaster cast, itchy, heavy and cumbersome; the advice for coping with the itching was to pour surgical spirit down inside but this only worked for an itch close to the top of the plaster, so I developed my own method, frowned on by authority as so much of my personalised way of coping tended to be, and that was an old plastic belt with a small buckle that I could thread from the top and then pull through, the buckle an excellent provider of relief.

A shameful incident took place during one of the tiresome plaster cast episodes when Mum caught me up in her arms away from the friends I was playing with to take me indoors; I was embarrassed to be grabbed away like that with my friends there to see my humiliation and decided enough was enough. I struggled and fought her, unfortunately catching her in the face with my plaster encased leg. This was accidental but I then had to suffer hearing her tell all and sundry that I had kicked her in the face. The stubbornness of my nature meant I could not bring myself to deny her interpretation of events, although I do so now. It was an accident.

Walking for more than a short distance was out owing to the heavy cast and was not possible immediately after a bleed anyway so Mum asked Old Egghead if a wheelchair could be provided as a standby after a bleed and for longer distance travel. The answer was no as if I used a wheelchair at all I would want to stay in it all the time. Foolish Egghead, I hated being restricted in any way and when out to play I would take my trusty footstool and sit down for a rest every few hundred yards. Friends and I would go on expeditions to 'The New River' when arguments as to who I had delegated to carry the stool developed, this worked well when mooching round the neighbourhood but not when going with Mum to the Co-Op for instance. So Mum solved the problem by hiring from the Red Cross an old attendant pushed wheelchair, which we kept for many years. I did not use the chair all the time but remain grateful to Mum and the Red Cross for giving me the opportunity to visit places and go for long walks from which I would otherwise have been excluded.

Grandad gone, his dog Billy gone, my brother married and living with his in-laws, the Atkins', even my little girlfriend Elizabeth gone, moved to another house a few streets away. The living-room seemed hot and airless and I would have to go to the back-door and fling it open to get some air and cool off, this was not popular with my parents but very necessary to me, the rush of cool fresher air, remember all the coal-fires before the clean air act, was a tremendous relief. In the day-time the rooms were dark and depressing and not as I'd imagined and hoped to return to when my three year banishment was over.

Chapter 24

I'd had similar negative feelings on returning home from hospital pre-Corley but these would be short-lived, now it took time to overcome the stifled feelings but I very quickly saw the unnaturally dim daylight level as acceptable.

The neighbours remained the same, apart from Elizabeth and family who'd disappointingly moved a short distance away. Brian now had a most remarkable dog, Rover, so adept at slipping his collar and making his way out of the garden to roam near and far that I would see him two or three miles away running about with other dogs on many a green space; I'd watched him crossing roads, not for him the way some dogs ignored the traffic and ran across just as they chose, indeed, running about in the roads, Rover would stop at the kerb, look both ways and only cross when it was safe to do so

On the other side of us the Turralls, Mr and Mrs, their grown-up children Lance and Pat, had been joined by Willow, the Cat and Tiger the dog.

Our front doors were only a couple of feet apart and everyone who came to either door would be startled by Tiger suddenly appearing in the bay-window next to the door barking loudly. Occasionally it wouldn't be Tiger, but Lance, barking and snarling, such fun, and whenever I came up the path a most delicious smell would come wafting from their house, percolating coffee!

Brian and I took up our friendship again but as he was now a schoolboy it could not be quite the same, he had other friendships to maintain and was able to be more active than I who was burdened down with the calliper, nevertheless when his parents went out at the weekend Brian, Rover and me would play together next door with Mum keeping an eye on us. I don't remember what we did only that we were together and Rover would chase his tail if you said 'cheeeese' elongating the middle 'e' sound, and would rush around looking up in the air growling if you did the same thing with the word 'flies'.

Ronnie and I never renewed our friendship; I think both of us were somewhat embarrassed when we met up again. David I spent time with occasionally but this was usually arranged by our respective mothers.

David was always a very good boy, which could not be said of me, and quite unadventurous. I remember the feelings of frustration and disgust on a snowy winter's day when he on his side of the road and I on mine were making snow-balls and I challenged him to a snowball battle and he refused. He was obeying orders not to do anything that might cause me a bleed, but I reassured him that snowballs would not be a problem. I'd been smacked in the mouth by a hard-driven tennis ball at Corley with no consequences apart from the immediate shock but he couldn't be persuaded and I went off in a huff. What he couldn't know was that I chose him for snowballing because most other kids would not hesitate to mould their snowballs round a stone just to see if I would bleed.

Jim had also returned from Corley and I went to his place very often during the first year or thereabouts. Parties at Jim's I remember most of all, there was a lad from across the street who put on a show of 'magic' on one occasion and I would always be asked to sing and be given money by the older relatives. Less happily someone always remarked how wonderful God's works were as He compensated 'them' with a talent to make up for 'their' illness. As I thought of myself as a free individual, never part of any 'them' and the theory that God had decided to allow haemophilia into my life but add in, just to make it up to me, a talent for singing was anathema to me. Come to think of it, two older ladies were responsible for these utterances on God and his mercy and these same ladies were convinced that if only I came to their church, The Little Bethel, I would be cured of my affliction by the laying on of hands. Mum being willing to try anything and having a belief in God it was arranged and off we went me in my Red-Cross wheelchair.

How we got to the other side of the city centre I don't know but with the four of us getting nearer to the church, one of the two ladies asked to be allowed to push the wheelchair, she seemed excited and as we reached the church which was on the other side of the road, headed us to the kerb and unceremoniously dropped the front wheels down onto the tarmac. Now, if you have ever assisted a push-chair or a wheelchair down a kerb you will know that you pull back and let the rear wheels descend first. If you suddenly drop the front wheels down from the kerb.........I was decanted into the road so suddenly and was so angry that the poor lady's ears were assaulted by the choicest of the ranker part of my vocabulary with the addition of the information that she was stupid. As usual everyone asked if I was alright, luckily my head had not come into contact with the road or I might well have been in serious need of God's ever- loving mercy within a very short time. The several aches and pains the experience left me with might or might not have developed into a bleed or heavy bruising and I would be on tenterhooks until the next day, so once again, 'was I alright?' I'd have to wait and see. We did eventually get into the church, hands were laid on, my haemophilia did not respond, and I heard a whisper that my bad language and general naughtiness was the reason. As no bleed occurred from my startling contact with the macadam, perhaps that was a miracle? No I'd suffered much worse trauma without bleeding, and much, much less with serious consequences, a pattern that continued into adulthood.

After another party at the Cooper's my wheelchair which had been folded-up in the hall had to be resurrected into a usable state, this wheelchair folded down with all four wheels on the ground and to open for use the front was held down by a foot while pulling on the back then two clips one on each side were snapped into position to stabilise it. Someone rushed to do the job saying let me do it and when I sat in the thing, the clips not having been secured, it suddenly closed up, folding me in half, trapping me as meat in a wheelchair sandwich, again I made with the bad language and my favourite other words, stupid and idiot. It required many hands making light work to retrieve the situation and with some holding down the front and others pulling back I obtained release.

Jim was sent to Ventnor, Isle of Wight for his asthma as the air coming off the sea was supposed to help, as was his stay at Corley with the fresh air that we all benefited from. What it meant to me was that one of my best friends was removed from me and forced me to look to my other friends. It may have been before Jim went away that time, events around our friendship are a little mixed and vague, but he sent me, via Mum, a working model of a guillotine made in part from pieces of a pencil sharpener and geometry set, a macabre instrument that could decapitate a Plasticene man with great efficiency and an amount of realism supplied by red food colouring. Two other gifts he sent me, the first a toy Land-Rover with a superstructure of Plasticene which turned it into a sort of miniature caravan.

It's shaming that I don't believe I ever thanked him for these presents or went to see him for that matter, with hindsight this appears to be another instance of not wanting to be involved with anyone who was going to be here one minute and gone the next, did I know perhaps that he would be going away to the Isle of Wight and did this influence me, I was still, after all, a child. He came home again but was then sent to Davos, Switzerland by the Red Cross for the mountain air.

Other friendships developed with Elsie, Elaine McCalman, Robin's young sister, and my cousin Peter, always known as Pete and his friends Denise and Sheila.

Pete, Sheila , and Denise had started clubs which as far as I remember included just those three, I was invited to join and did so but the clubs seemed very tame to me and apart from reading Enid Blyton stories and looking for four-leaf clovers didn't appear to have any other purpose. The Clover Club could not be joined unless one had found a four-leaved clover and I soon found that this elusive leaf was almost impossible to find and was disgusted to learn the trick of finding one, this was accomplished by the expedient use of the thumb nail to split a leaflet in two. The other club was the Sunny Stories Club, but the stories in the magazine were unexciting to one who had chased girls all around vast playing fields to add their hair to a coup-stick. Eventually I became deeply attached to Denise and we spent a lot of time together.

Chapter 25

She told me that she hadn't known there was a boy living just across the road and I explained that this was probably because I had been at Corley for three years.

Pete lived with his parents, Uncle Bob and Aunt Doris, his brother, older than both of us, also named Bob and two cats Timmy and Tibby. Uncle Bob was Dad's younger brother and business partner and the relationship was not without friction. The simmering resentment Dad felt for his younger brother did not stop them sitting over pints of beer at the local pub, the Devonshire Arms. If your father drank there then it was possible to enter the garden and tap on the window on spying him, this several kids did with the proviso that if done too frequently the barman would open the window and tell you 'Yer Dad says go home!' But used with restraint a few raps on the window would lead to Dad buying you a drink and the barman opening a window behind the bar and handing it out. The system held the possibility of being painful for me as on one occasion Mum, when I was being particularly irritating, told me to go down to the Devon and see if Dad wanted anything to do with me. I went, I tapped, I saw Dad look out of the corner of his eye and then astonishingly take another sip of his beer. Surely he wouldn't ignore me? I tapped harder and again he looked sideways while ostensibly looking towards the bar, devastating, but Uncle Bob turned and looked, spoke to him and Dad gave me a look at last and ordered me a drink. My confidence had been shattered and the only time I went to the window again was with Pete when we would both knock and Uncle Bob would buy both of us a drink.

I spent many hours over the road at Pete's house in the early years after my return from Corley, playing indoors or in the back garden which was fairly standard apart from the Anderson shelter I'd spent a night in as a baby which now stood above ground and was used as a shed, this in itself being a fairly standard fate when shelter from bombs was no longer felt to be necessary.

Aunt Doris was a cheerful person with a way of smiling and listening with her head held to one side, she was invariably nice to me although I can't think of any great deeds of affection or, more unusually for me, disapprobation. To avoid confusion I shall refer to the older Bob as Uncle Bob and his son, the younger as Bob.

Bob was some years older than me and attended grammar school, and like all schoolboys had his fair share of problems. He suffered badly from migraine at times and what could you add to migraine that would make matters worse? Hay fever! I can't imagine what it must feel like sneezing a dozen times one after the other when assailed by awful head pain.

Our noisy games always seemed to spill into the hall and if Bob was wrestling with his migraine in his darkened bedroom this must have been torture, after a while a shout of 'Shut up!' would echo down the stairs, Pete would giggle and I would be mortified that I'd made matters worse for Bob and resolve to keep the noise down, not much chance of that, we quickly forgot in the throes of imaginative play and again would come the exasperated cry. At this point or perhaps the third command we would issue forth into the garden, entry, street or over The Dump.

Bob, Pete and Aunt Doris were Jehovah's Witnesses, Bob eventually becoming disassociated. I have no idea when Aunt Doris became involved with the witnesses, but assume that she led Bob and Pete into it, nothing derogatory meant, following her belief for the rest of her life as does Peter to this day. I once studied with them for a time but quickly became disillusioned with the whole thing, as study meant reading a passage and then answering multiple choice questions. Each answer would have a sensible choice, the correct one, a semi-sensible choice and a really silly one. My perverse nature ensured that my preferred choice was the silly answer, it was always obvious which was correct, but although tempted I withstood the temptation out of respect for my aunt and cousin, eventually saying I didn't want to participate any further. I did attend the Kingdom Hall once but found it tedious in the extreme and the people too good for me, at least on the surface.

Uncle Bob was not a witness and this must have led to much difficulty and distress, not spoken of but acknowledged in whispers by various members of the greater family. On arriving back from holiday he would bring me a gift, once a cooked lobster which never got eaten, which could have been my fault, wanting to keep it. During another holiday a tin of clotted cream arrived, a Cornish delicacy, sent through the post; my parents brought it in to Cleaver. On opening I was surprised to see a crust on the cream and Mum and Dad said it was off and I mustn't eat it. 'Typical of him to send something like that through the post he might have known it would go off.' says Dad. 'We'll get rid of it.' Next visiting day Mum tells me we put some salt in and it was just like butter your Dad had it on his Sandwiches. I believe the above incidents were prompted by jealousy, not aimed at me but Uncle Bob, depriving me was coincidental, if they truly believed the cream was off why add salt and eat it? A trivial matter no doubt of that but indicative of the negative way Dad looked on his brother.

If it hadn't been for Uncle Bob I would never have visited the circus, he came and asked could he take me as they were going, my parents agreement was a bit of a surprise as fairs and circuses caused Mum to worry as she was sure all sorts of diseases could be caught there, but I was at last going to the circus.

It was distressing to be picked up by Uncle Bob and carried in his arms to the front of the queue where special pleading got us in first, not that I minded getting to the front, I was already worried about standing there for so long, but his describing me as 'a spastic' while short and easy for the attendant to understand mortified me, still I admired the way he'd dealt with the situation and his appreciation of my problem with queuing, something that plagued me most of my life, being better able to walk than stand.

Two incidents I shall never forget, the first a deed I have remained grateful for to this day and the second which puzzles me even now.

One evening Uncle Bob came over and told us he was taking Pete to the library and asked would I like to go, always ready for a trip out, off we went. Kingsway Library wasn't far to travel and we went in his car, once there and surrounded by books, it looked like heaven and when asked if I would like to join I was very happy to do so. Library tickets were issued and I chose two books there and then, The Tigers of Trengganu by A. Locke, first published 1954, beautifully written, an excellent start to my library adventures, I have no memory of the other book but I read, over the next few months, everything on big game subjects that Kingsway held and what a boon the library proved, no more wondering if I was going to run out of reading material and have to cope with a bleed without the distraction technique of reading.

I Learned, and continue to learn so much from libraries. The two greatest gifts I ever had, my library tickets, and the complete works of Dickens. My gratitude for these has never faltered. I wish I could tempt myself to leave Uncle Bob in fully generous mode but an unfortunate incident must be my last mention.

I was ill in bed, when Mum came in carrying two large volumes, bound in green leatherette with gold lettering, unfortunately my memory of what the lettering read is gone. A lady who lived a few doors down the street, Mrs Bowistow was moving to Cornwall or maybe Devon and had asked Mum to 'Give these to your lad'. I couldn't have been more pleased, both volumes had many illustrations, both photographs and etchings, the first being full of antiquities such as stone circles, packhorse bridges and the like and the second of folk events, maypoles, well-dressing, various teams of dancers and so on. I already had great interest in pre-history and bygone things and ways so was delighted to have these books. Sometime later I was in bed recovering yet again and reading these books when Uncle Bob came up to see me 'What have you there, Derek.' 'Books Mrs Bowistow gave me'. Bombshell! No, he told me those belong to Bob and despite my protests took them away with him. I was astonished and embarrassed and when I told Mum what had happened she did nothing about it, this incident has puzzled me ever since, did Mrs Bowistow make a mistake, had she borrowed them from Bob and meant Mum to return them to him, not very likely, but possible. Had Mum lifted them from Uncle Bob's home and given them to me, an act of thievery straight out of fantasy and even more unlikely, or had Uncle Bob been mistaken or even stolen them thinking them too good and valuable for me, this latter while unthinkable to me was what my father suggested when I mentioned it to him a couple of years later by which time Uncle Bob had a new name as far as Mum and Dad were concerned 'Big 'ead' was how they referred to him.

Pete and I saw less and less of each other as time went by but at first we played together an awful lot. I would go over to his house and take my fort and soldiers after he acquired a fort and soldiers too and both would be set up and populated with soldiers and a battle would begin. His fort had integral gun turrets from which he rained down spent matches and I had a model field gun which was more accurate but more difficult to load, neither of us liked it when any of our troops were 'killed' and elaborate supplementary fortifications constructed from books would quickly be erected so that the outcome was always stalemate. Transferring to the back garden and a pile of sand that gradually spread over part of the lawn we would make this the area where toy cowboys and Indians took over from the toy soldiers and rode around avoiding each other, during one prolonged bout of non-engagement Pete had a call of nature and had to go indoors making me promise not to do anything until he returned. Alas, this was an opportunity not to be lightly ignored and I quickly constructed a slit trench, put in those of my 'men' who held rifles ready to fire and covered it with a strip of cardboard and a light sprinkling of sand, when Pete returned he looked all around and decided all was as he left it. Then a number of my horsemen galloped close to his position and out came his to chase them away, oh unkind perfidious Derek they were led into an ambush.

Chapter 26

The usual way these games were played was with a commentary, on this occasion thus. D: My men tease your men by riding close to them. P: then my men come out from behind the hill and chase them away. D: My men who have ridden a long way to get there have tired horses. P: my men are getting closer to yours and have shot one off his horse, there that one, yes. D: My men in the trench open fire and kill or wound all your men. P: (in tears) that's not fair I asked you not to do anything, Mum, Derek's cheating! This taught me that my talent for skulduggery was still intact and that triumph often came, when it came, with the knowledge that one had indeed broken the rules of the game. I knew many adults who went in for cheating and breaking the law so I chose to forgive, as after many other nefarious deeds, myself.

Denise was, by now, definitely my girlfriend. I enjoyed every moment we spent together, the ever possible anger never reared its head with her and if I slipped into it with others in front of her I felt shame. I could see a future at last, the two of us together against the world's hostility.

One cold day Denise was shivering, why I never invited her into the warmth of the house is lost to me now, but I had hidden a box of matches and we made a warming fire on The Dump and sat against it, this was a very well controlled fire inside a square of bricks. All was warm and cosy, with just the two of us but inevitably idiotic boys came begging for a light and I reluctantly gave them access, within ten minutes they went from making fires similar to mine but with no skill at all, to trying to catch the grass alight and chasing each other with burning sticks.

I was about to say that we should put out our fire and go when a policeman turned up, obviously alerted by a 'concerned' neighbour and Denise shot off leaving me to face the law. Momentarily I felt put out by her precipitate disappearance but quickly realised the sense behind it. It was well known that I was a naughty boy, accepted by her parents as her friend but if she got into trouble with the law through me her father would have seen to it that we were kept apart. The policeman asked who had the matches and in my disgust at allowing the others to spoil things, I said me and when he asked for them I threw them at him as hard as I could, I poured the earth and sand I had ready over the fire and he asked me where I lived, which was just down the bank and across the entry, and he took me home, we entered through the back-door and, what luck, Mum had gone to the shops, so he told me not to light any more fires and took the matches with him.

The loss of the matches was a severe blow as they had taken ingenuity to acquire. Mum had long since asked the local shopkeepers not to serve me with matches, the mothers of local kids, who on several days had been cured of their boredom by the making of chips, cooked over an open fire, when I would ask one to get a frying pan another fat or oil and another salt and potatoes, had complained to Mum that their kids were well-fed at home and little Jimmy hadn't eaten his dinner etc. and other Mums and Dads objected to fire ships floating down the ditch in winter. I couldn't swear that I would never indulge again, hence the ban. A life without matches was not acceptable to me so I hatched a plan.

I hung around Mum, getting under her feet and asking questions she couldn't answer until, judging the time to be right, I asked could I go to the shop for her? She was astonished to have me ask such a question but the softening up by previous skilled irritation made the offer one she felt she must accept. She gave me money and a list of two or three items, not too much as she didn't want me to wrench my arms and cause a bleed and out the door I went with confidence in my plan. In the local grocery store I read from my list the two or three items, checking it minutely each time and casually added a box of matches, the assistant accepted this, I left with Mum's items in the bag and my item safely pocketed. Mum didn't ask about the receipt so no need for my prepared innocent answer that I didn't know you were supposed to keep it, which would have been believed because of my lack of experience in shopping, and the change seemed right as everyone knew the prices just down the street were higher than the Co-op.

Reader, I had my matches, an essential tool of the trade as ideas man to others who relied on my penchant for suggesting new and interesting things to do. During the summer, school holidays left them bored long before the end and they would tell me they were bored and ask what we could do, I'd tell them to let me think and they'd sit quietly while I thought, there would always be one to break my mental tergiversating and repeat 'I'm bored' and someone who'd reply, 'Shut up! He's thinking aint he?' and as I was always about when work left by my tutor had been completed I could prepare tomahawk blades, for instance, by shaping bits of slate to an elongated triangle and a ground sharp edge for my pals to attach to greenwood sticks. All this ceased during term time once I started school and was never to be resurrected.

Stan and Vi had two pet shops in Birmingham, one a lock-up and the other they lived over. We went to stay with them for a holiday, which in retrospect seems a little odd but at the time I accepted. The disappointment came when the monkey I'd expected to see sitting at the breakfast table eating with the Barretts and attired in a fez had been sold, the other pets were fascinating however and the smell of sawdust and doggy-biscuits very satisfactory, the green meat however was revolting, and I learnt that it was dyed green because it was unfit for human consumption. It seemed strange to me at the time that the Barrett's had two pet shops full of fauna of all descriptions yet kept a dog of their own, a kind of coals-to-Newcastle feeling although today it would not seem strange to me at all, I remember the oddness.

Vi Barrett, Auntie Vi as I was encouraged to call her, loved a pop-song of the time, with truly horrible lyrics that set my teeth on edge, I have no memory of the singer's name but the song was called The Story of Tina and the first few words were:

The story of Tina began in the springtime
When Tina was sweet seventeen.

These words are burned into my memory as if with a branding iron, and if they were mawkish then both the amorous career of Tina and the rest of the song were on the beginning of a skid to the bottom. The other memory, also musical to an extent, associated with the holiday is one that has haunted me ever since.

At the time, the pop industry was centred on what was known as Tin-Pan-Alley and this horror mostly produced dubious ballads such as that rubbished above and novelty songs. The Barrett's, Mum, Dad and me went to a large pub somewhere near Birmingham where a midlands band was playing, I had to stay in the kitchen, or so I was told, and if I saw a policeman to call them, suddenly a small window opened and a policeman's hat bobbed up and down outside on a stick, turning as it did so in a grotesque fashion and then disappeared. Shortly after, Uncle Stan and Dad plus one or two other characters came into the kitchen and the question was asked, had I seen a policeman, no, I had however seen a policeman's helmet on a stick. They looked at one another and shook their heads.

This was not the thing that has worried me ever since that night however, I was asked to sing, and sang one of the current novelty songs, the bandleader, it turned out was looking for a mascot, most of these dance bands had such a thing, and if a boy he would be dressed in the band's uniform and would be with them on stage and get to sing one or two novelty songs during the performance, the job was offered to me and I turned it down. I loved singing and entertaining but........

I was astonished that my haemophilia was not a consideration, and these were adults? Adults were supposed to have the capacity to take decisions based on logical evaluation of the possible actions and consequences of any new suggestion and act accordingly, I could not have explained that at the time but I could see for myself what was almost a certain outcome barring a miracle. Here's the scene: I say yes, I get measured and a uniform is provided, someone is sent to collect me for a gig, I could be starting a bleed and would then have to decide whether or not to reveal it or to go through with it hoping that I'd last out until the end of the gig and my return home, or I might develop a bleed when somewhere with the band, miles away, as they played all over the midlands and someone would then have to take me home. I was bitterly disappointed that I had to turn down the opportunity but even more disappointed that no-one had bothered to protect me from making such a decision on my own.

My father's disappointment was never spoken of, but I could see how puzzled he was by my refusal to take a step that many other kids of my age would have dreamed of. Shirley Abicair, an Australian singer and zither player would, a couple of years or so after appear on our first television, and one day Dad turned to me and pointedly remarked, 'She's made her parents very happy.' this said he turned back to the screen with his lips clamped firmly together in a straight line and I knew the phrase was a rebuke. Now that prophylactic treatment of haemophilia has progressed there would be no need for me to refuse such an offer, but where's the lost young boy, to misquote Housman.

Back at home the games, the popular games we played, some of which were frowned on by adults and one I never played being concerned for my ankles, took up a great deal of my time. The game I was forced to avoid I found very attractive but knew from watching the others that it could easily bring disaster to me. This was less of a game than a creative use of scrap materials and fun, being the making and using of 'stilts' made from tin cans and string, two holes would be made in the bottom of a couple of golden syrup or similar tins, then a loop of string was threaded through the holes and knotted at each end, the same process repeated on the other can, leaving two cans on two loops of string.

Chapter 27

These were the stilts and by standing on the cans and pulling the loops of string tight, it was possible to lift each foot and walk forward with the cans held firmly onto the soles of the shoes. A rise in stature of approximately six inches was achieved, the less desirable outcome was a loud clank at every step, perturbing to the hearer if the perpetrators were hidden from view, and I observed many a dangling lower jaw and gestures of slight alarm as onlookers awaited a sight of the clanking 'thing' approaching from round the corner. This was at least an amusing happenstance for an observer of all and everything and I chose to watch as closely as possible, my reward being the times when several stilt-walkers walked down to the local shops and paraded about until driven away by angry shop-keepers when they hurried off on their stilts and the clanging and clashing became furious and battle-like, and nothing could be heard above the din.

Bows and arrows was one of the games that I could play but this was not without parental interference with dire warnings about lost eyes, which of course were never heeded and never happened but a kid who refused to take precautions against the possibility would quickly find himself isolated, his bow confiscated and destroyed. To allay the fears of parents I came up with the idea of making one arrow with a padded end, and making sure that this was the one you were caught using, thus avoiding the ritual admonitions as parents floated by on their inscrutable and boring missions.

Fag-cards or cigarette cards were often traded and searched for outside the Devon and the shops, and a couple of games were played with them. The simplest involved taking turns to skim cards and try to land on each other's when the cards yours rested on were then added to your cache, the other involved standing a number of cards against the wall and skimming in turn to knock them over, the winner took that card and any that had missed the target card.

The most dangerous game was a nuisance to play in the street as one was constantly warned of the possibility of death by dart. Not darts as the Darts Regulation Authority would recognise the term but darts made from a short stick, say nine inches long, sharpened at one end and with a nail driven in at an angle and extra weight added, ideally with lead taped on or perhaps just a bunch of tape, the other end of the stick would be split in cruciform pattern and a flight, made of cardboard or plastic affixed. Another, shorter piece of stick was fashioned into a slingshot/launcher by affixing a powerful elastic loop, and the nail sticking out of the dart used to anchor the elastic, the launcher held in one hand and the dart pulled back against the tension of the elastic and released, the object was to see whose dart would climb the highest. The danger was on re-entry as the darts would plummet down as though fired from a cross-bow and if several had been fired at once it could be hard to dodge them. The only accident that I saw however was when the elastic broke free at one end and flew round onto the hand or wrist of the aimer. Darts were usually played on the dump, as darting passers-by would not have been tolerated and besides it might be someone we knew or who perhaps could be of use at some other time. The difficulty that the dump threw up was that the vegetation was varied and unkempt so a dart had to be watched very closely to ascertain where it had come to rest, much time was wasted in this way and occasionally some less than honest kid would find and conceal it and hope to make off with it later when its owner had given up the search, a pointless exercise as everyone knew whose it was and the thief could never use it.

The Dump or, as other kids from farther up the street and from the streets around knew it, The Tip in either case it deserves an initial capital letter, was a superb unofficial children's facility. I know the name evokes a horrible waste of rotting muck and swarms of gulls but even allowing for the glamour years can bring to any prospect, this was heaven, an unregulated, adult free adventure playground, that for home owners was an eyesore bringing down property values, but for us kids provided an opportunity to escape to play and to learn valuable lessons concerning co-operation, tolerance at least some of the time, responsibility for our actions, leadership for some and how to construct from found materials.

Physically The Dump was an area of land between the row of houses on your right if facing away from the Devonshire Arms up the hill towards the allotments which split Sewell Highway in two, this was bounded on the other side by a ditch then farmland and another field known as the cornfield, because it had once within memory held a crop of wheat. The Dump had been acquired by the city council during the blitz to take the tons of rubble from bombed out houses and by consequence of so much being dumped was raised above ground level in places about nine foot, grass, patches of nettles and an assortment of weeds and/or wild flowers moved in and a landscape with ups and downs, mini plains and hills soon developed. There were two bomb craters, one much deeper than the other, and when the other kids were bored one of my ideas was to do reverse mountain climbing and with a 'borrowed' clothes line for rope, suitable sticks for ice-axes we slid to the bottom of the deepest crater and made our way diagonally up the treacherous slope of Holey Mountain with many a slip and slide.

The ditch that bounded the dump would dry up in the summer but at times made a very fine stream to be bridged or dammed, or in one place where a flattened area made it possible, a delta of small channels and larger ponds could be made. Originally this ditch had joined another running across from it and this dived underground into a large diameter pipe, fortunately for us, protected by strong metal bars. This tunnel if not sealed by bars would surely have had the more intrepid down there on a caving expedition.

Hide and seek, kisses and maybe more in the hollows, kite flying, the ebb and flow of top dog status and among the many little gangs, each with a leader, alliances and battles, all were ours, no supervision, no wet-blanket interference. And then there were the tracks we constructed down the steep slope of the banked up Dump ending in the entry behind our houses.

These tracks were similar to bob-sleigh courses at the winter Olympics, with curves and straights, and banked sharp curves but ours were for Dinky Toys and other model cars which when sent from the top built up great speed by the bottom. At first every attempt ended in disaster and no-one had a car, racing or otherwise, reach the bottom still on four wheels, but with suggestions of where the curve needed banking and the shortening of straights and many a 'discussion' about whose contribution should be acted on, eventually the perfect track would be constructed and whether or not your car reached the bottom safely and quickly was only down to your skill in placement and the degree of push-off at the start. Starting two together was exciting but it was rare to get two finishers and more often than our optimism allowed neither would finish. The tracks were always short lived as they were constructed around paths up from the entry and onto the dump, and when we came back next day we would find them ruined as someone had used the path in the way originally intended.

When I first came home from Corley squatters lived in the old army huts still adorning the field beyond The Dump and Cornfield, years after the war had finished, and these people were looked on with great suspicion by our parents. Pretty soon the squatters were gone and the camp pulled down so that the only person left as a magnet for prejudice was the 'nudist' who lived on his own land in a caravan on the private allotments which, until compulsorily purchased, split Sewell Highway in half.

These allotments were wonderful with cinder paths in a grid and small businesses amid the more ordinary vegetable growing enterprises, including a pig-farm, Bott's Nursery with a great many greenhouses, and Mrs Busby's rag and bone enterprise. Mrs Busby was a well-known character who pushed an old pram around the area 'collecting' rag and bone and any other scrap she could fit into the pram. She was always followed by a couple of dogs, my memory tells me they were bull terriers though of this I'm not sure, I say dogs but they were in fact bitches which always had well-used teats hanging down so maybe she sold puppies as well.

The naturist who lived on his allotment often came down the hill on his bike in just a pair of shorts and you would have thought he was wearing nothing to hear the clucked warnings by our fat, hair-curlered and pinafored 'mother-hens' as they gathered their offspring around them and warned once more to keep away from the allotments. They used to tell one another how terrible it was that he should take off all his clothes for anyone to see and how wrong it was for the kiddies. I'd almost definitely seen the man in my Big, Giant Dream anyway.

Chapter 28

Dreams played a big part in my life, not dreams of what I would do with my life when grown to a man but actual sleeping dreams.

Around the age of ten years I had a dream that influenced me throughout the rest of my childhood with the chief character appearing in other dreams right up to somewhere between my thirtieth and fortieth year and I have retained the important details to this day.

A crowd of people including everyone I know are swarming down into a pedestrian subway in the city centre trying to escape falling bombs. I was swept along with the crowd, until a smaller tunnel opened on the left and almost like being caught by an eddy in a swift flowing river I found myself impelled into it with my family and friends all moved on by the crush my mother looking at me reproachfully but I knowing that this was the way for me to go, and I went. Far down the tunnel two other figures hurried along in the distance and as the tunnel curved I lost sight of them. Eventually I emerged into a beautiful meadow dotted with trees, with a broad river with moored to the bank a three-quarter-sized sailing vessel, not a model but not very large; I mounted the gang-plank and stepped aboard causing the vessel to dip slightly. Two figures stood diagonally across from me gazing down over the side at the water; on the right a tall man, bearded with long hair, a fur waistcoat and a horned head-dress, on his left a girl with long, straight, blond hair dressed in a one piece white tunic that reached the ground. The girl turned her head, smiled and made room for me to come and stand between them; this I did and both pointed at the water.

What may or may not be a standard dream, and indeed I can easily connect the elements to my life and memories at the time, becomes more difficult to accept and if a reader is sceptical or even repelled so be it.

What all three of us were now looking at was, moving from right to left as though scrolling, a pageant and an explanation of events and people and my part in the interconnected nature of everything and everyone, through all time. Revelation after revelation, so much information, including matters I could not or did not know much, if anything, about. The flow was very fast and try as I might it was impossible to hold onto anything specific as startling fact and explanation raced past.

How long the dream took I don't know but I continued to struggle to bring up to the surface at least some of what I'd learned. It never happened. I believe, though cannot prove, that as hinted the knowledge exists deep in memory and surfaces at times in images that erupt unbidden. No long list of instances just one; I saw in my mind the vials of factor ix long before they were developed. The general size and the size of label, and what the contents would look like.

The girl in my dream made appearance after appearance throughout the rest of my childhood and on until my late thirties, pulling me toward her and leaving me longing as she ran from me. In my mind she equated with Denise, she looked like Denise or the essence of her and something feminine in the universal. Eventually she ran no more, I caught her and we rolled together down a grassy bank as she laughed, not at me but with joy that I finally understood how easy it could be and we merged, became one, no, not sexually; two separate halves had become one and my unintentional reluctance to allow the fulfilling of this desired condition was what had made her run.

Chapter 29

But to return the notorious nudist; needless to say the poor man had taken every precaution to avoid the little innocents seeing him with a metal fence and a deep hedge, the only way to be frightened or outraged was to burrow through the hedge, oh the prejudice of the petty artisans, factory workers and their wives, victims of their own ordinariness.

A great many of my relatives we never saw, and I think this was a policy of Dad's, I can only hope that his reticence had nothing to do with finding my medical condition awkward. There are so many who only mean a name and one or two anecdotes to me. Dad's sister my aunt Win died not long before I was born, of quinsy whatever quinsy might be, leaving three children, Alan, Rose and John and husband Jim Sproul. Rose and my brother were great friends, being cousins of roughly the same age; Alan the eldest brother I met on numerous occasions but recall little of him except he had a wife, Margaret and one son Mark. Rose worked as a land girl either towards the end of the war or just after and married Pete Bennett who hailed from deepest rural Warwickshire, Bidford-on-Avon.

The Cooper's seemed more like family to me, I loved visiting their house which was better appointed and without the constant harping on and sniping at relatives that I found distressing at home; Syd and Violet his wife, my aunt and uncle and, in Mum's case, Gran all criticised with every action and remark freely disparaged.

The Cooper's had three cats Patch, Monty and another, whose name escapes me, then a kitten turned up, four cats were too many and Mum allowed herself to be persuaded to bring the kitten, now practically grown, home for me. I named her Dinky but didn't have much time to love her as she was got at by a local cat which had a very strangely screwed up face, possibly the result of some kind of accident, this cat was called The Phantom Tom by Mum and had been hanging around the garden awaiting his opportunity. He sprang on Dinky one day and there was a terrible fight as she wasn't ready for a Tom. Fur flew and shit flew as she was terrified, I ran at them and frightened him off. In spite of my vigilance the inevitable happened and Dinky, little more than a kitten was pregnant, this signalled her end. Mum took her 'To a farm, where she'll be better off.' This euphemism meant destroyed, put down, put to sleep. No chance of neutering, that would have cost money, kittens tended to be drowned in a bucket of water when quite young a process repeated over and over in some cases. I knew what had really taken place, the RSPCA had premises quite near and she'd been killed, disposed of. In later years I found out that the method of dealing with unwanted pets that they used was to put them in a cage with a metal floor and throw a switch, electrocuting them for the crime of being born.

I hated and blamed The Phantom Tom and when I heard it had been hit by a car I went into its back garden to torment it, but when I saw it lying on the back door-step of its home in an obviously bad way with blood too, I felt sorry for it and slipped away. I did nothing to help it, and can only point out that I was a child of only, perhaps, ten and still blamed it for the loss of Dinky. Later I saw how Gertie Cooper was a little responsible for trusting the cat to my mother, but that Mum herself was the main culprit for not at least trying to get Dinky fixed, most especially as I overheard her saying to someone 'She was a dirty little thing anyway, she liked it.' This puzzled me at first until I realised she meant Phantom's impregnation. I'm so glad neither of my parents saw fit to offer me sex education!

Brian went to live with his Gran after his parents split up, his Dad and Rover staying on for a time until one day Mum told me that Rover had been taken to stay on a farm, I knew this was a euphemism for put-down as she had said the same when she had my kitten destroyed. Dad told me that it was a shame Rover had gone because he was going to say we would have him, I despised Dad for saying it as I doubted it was true and anyway he'd had plenty of time to arrange it if he'd really intended to; I have never forgotten or, regrettably, forgiven either parent for denying me my pets. Not that I stopped loving my parents but the mistrust of Mum because of her being the one who took me into hospital, and my slow disenchantment with Dad was hard enough for me to deal with.

Joey my budgie, I had later. Bert Roberts, Elsie's Dad bred budgies and gave me a young bird. She was lovely and enjoyed being out of her cage flying round and playing with me. I would come downstairs in the morning and lie on the floor with my leg in the air, she would land on my toe and as I lowered my leg to make a slope run down along my body, up onto my chin and kiss me on the lips then move on to my shoulder as I got to my feet. She had a toy in her cage which resembled the big wheel at a fairground, when I went up to her cage she would spin it with a flick of her beak and if I counted she would do it over and over, the same with another trick she learned she would hold onto the perch with one foot and the bars of the cage with the other and then push her head down between her legs and turn right round so that she faced the other way on the perch as she let go of the bars, this she also did over and over if I counted. She would beg, by holding onto the perch and vigorously flapping her wings, for a little of what I was eating and if suitable I'd give her a crumb or two and once when I was sucking a fruit gum she started and it made me laugh, the fruit gum was ejected from my mouth, shooting into her cage, she hopped onto the floor to search amongst the sand. We both frantically looked for the sweet, which was nowhere to be seen. She gave up and hopped back onto the perch, then looking uncomfortable lifted her wing and there was the missing fruit gum stuck to her body! Grabbing it in her beak she pulled it loose and slung it out of the cage. How I laughed then. I loved that bird!

Unfortunately she became another accessory in the battle between Mum and Gran who also had a budgie, a male and males are talkers, although the hen birds also imitate, the cock is the one noted for imitating speech. Gran would brag about how many words her bird knew, and say that the hens were what the breeders called throw-outs and that's why Mr Roberts had given Joey to me. Mum spent hours trying to get Joey to talk and blamed me for the failure, 'It's all that Nin talk you do that's stopped her.' What possessed me to start I don't know but I would say nin, nin, nin, in a high pitched voice and Joey and I would bob our heads up and down. Though Joey never 'talked' she could mimic Mum's cough which invariably consisted of three elements, more habitual than anything, also a knob on the cooker the turning of which produced a series of distinctive clicks. The rivalry was always intense between Mum and Gran and both the bird and I were mere pawns.

Mum would try to prevent me going out to play, her version was that Harry Parry had told her to keep me in and perhaps that was so, but it soon became difficult for her to achieve as my ingenuity was stimulated and anyway, bleeds could occur at any time, at any place and for very little reason. Some bleeds were called 'spontaneous' because no trauma could be associated with them, I never believed this as it only took a very small incident to start, for instance, a knee bleed, I don't know about trains and British Rail's 'wrong kind of snow' but a certain kind of snow, just a few centimetres deep with a hard surface but a lower layer that gave on walking when all the weight was on the leading foot causing a slight sudden increase in pressure often led to a bleed in my case. I am sure minute trauma such as these are to blame for ‘spontaneous’ bleeds.

My technique for getting out of the house: while Mum was busy in the kitchen/dining room I would take a book, tell her I was going to read it in the front room, hide behind the settee in the bay-window and read.

Chapter 30

Sometimes it took half-an-hour sometimes as much as three quarters but eventually she would call out to me and receiving no answer call more sharply and then burst into the front-room, look around and dash out of the front door with 'The little devil, he's got out'. Then came the tricky part, I had to get out from my hiding place, rush, calliper and all, through the house, out the back door, up the garden path, across the communal drive way always known as the entry and onto the dump where there were hollows, dens and a dry ditch to hide in. Meanwhile Mum, who never learned my secret, was traipsing up and down the street asking everyone she met if they had seen me and periodically calling my name, kids would come up to me and tell me she was looking for me and would look shocked when I replied that I knew. The ironic thing about all this is that in my haste to escape I may well have caused a bleed whereas if authority had left me alone it would not have happened.

Another curious spasm of ambitious parental enforcement would be the occasional abortive effort to make me eat. These always failed but there came the day when Mum decided, probably at Gran's insistence, delivered by Dad, to put her foot down. She set before me a large bowl of what she referred to as soup, when I say a large bowl I mean a pudding basin, this soup was always a dark brown colour, watery and with an oily surface and was in fact surplus gravy from cooking meat, water from boiled vegetables and a stock cube. Not that this tasted horrible, unusual yes but there was so much of it to dispose of. We both became stubborn in our rejection of the other's point of view and, tiresomely, she was reduced to the old and useless requirement that I should sit there until it was eaten. So I sat there and let my mind ramble until she had to go to the shops when she let me know that on coming back she wanted to see that it was gone. This suited me fine and once she was safely out of the way I took the basin up the garden and emptied it into the pig-swill bin, and on returning cleaned up the tell-tale signs that would have shown what had become of the 'soup'. Did she guess that I would pour it away if given the chance and break the stalemate, or did she genuinely expect me to pour it down my neck, I suspect the former.

Also annoying was being forced to go to bed before it was dark and when I could hear and see, by judicious curtain twitching, my mates still out enjoying the sunshine. This torture was another that Mum said Gran, via Dad, had stipulated, this may have been true or did Mum try to make me as resentful of Gran as she was? I would be instructed not to put the light on and even if I was not able to sleep I would at least be resting. No reading as this would 'strain my eyes', so I would wait for her to go downstairs and get out of bed, position myself so that I was close to the window with the corner of the curtain pulled back and read until the fading light made it impossible and then get back into bed and more often than not quickly fall asleep. But not before noticing a strange phenomenon that no-one seemed to understand when I mentioned it; in half-light I could see a small round object, internally agitated, on the wall and it seemed to move around the room along the dado strip. I understand now that this was happening within my eyesight but at the time it seemed to be independently mobile, obviously I was moving my eyes along the dado and this thing, whatever it was, was part of my vision. So much was it part of my visual world that I would say to people, 'You know that round thing that you can see sometimes.' and they never knew what on earth I was talking about. The phenomenon was not a solid spot but made up of constantly moving dots almost as though I could see an atom.

In retrospect my life at the time was a constant battle to maintain as much independence as possible, while acknowledging that at times I would have to submit to the ministrations of those whose duty was to help me, making up my own mind about what I should or should not do was most important, not obedience. One of Gran's strictures came directly to me when she told me I mustn't eat in my bedroom as it encouraged mice. I told her we didn't have mice in the house to encourage or discourage. 'You will if you eat in the bedroom, it encourages them.' I let it go as I loved Gran only acknowledging to myself that it made no sense at all. I was obliged to eat in my room if I was recovering from a bleed and what kind of mouse would enter the building, ignore the pantry and any crumbs available downstairs, on floor or tablecloth, and make its way up to my bedroom?

In those early post-Corley days Dad, who had started the business by then, would come in, eat and read the local newspaper then wash, change into a suit and go out to the local pub the Devonshire Arms, returning at 'chucking-out-time' and very soon after go to bed. Saturday he would go to the match if Coventry City had a home game, or go to the Devon early and sit with Uncle Bob, drinking. Sunday mornings meant a long lie in reading the papers, then a trip to see if anything had changed at the factory unit in French's yard, Godiva Street since the previous day, then dinner, then a nap which went on most of the afternoon, tea and then the Devon. This routine, or at least most of it went on all over the city, different pubs, different men but mostly the same dull performance which time had endowed with the aura of an adjunct necessary to the individual's sense of masculine verity.

I was sorry that I couldn't dredge up any enthusiasm for football, I just didn't care who had beaten who and one day I told him as it bothered me and I knew he cared desperately about Coventry City, I told him I didn't have any interest in football and he told me that when I was older I would, I thought he was wrong I didn't see how age had anything to do with the matter, but he was dead right, it happened and eventually I got myself a season ticket and the season after that we were promoted as champions of the second division to the first, now the

Premier League. I still buy a season ticket and hope to until I'm no longer capable of attending matches.

My education, after Corley was accomplished by a stint of home tuition and that was a wonderful time when I learned a great deal, and to which I owe much of my subsequent search for knowledge stimulated by the three tutors who took on the task so brilliantly.

The first teacher to come to the house was Mr Toogood, a lovely young man, whose teaching methods I don't recall but who led me further into the mysteries of English and Arithmetic. He didn't stay with the job for long, he worked in a local school by day and was not long married, but would come in the evenings and presumably leave me work to complete. On my birthday he brought me a Roy Rogers Album and his inscription read 'To Derek from his terrible teacher, Mr Toogood.' We heard that the baby that his wife was expecting had died and I expect he was devastated by this, I never heard what happened to him after that. Yet another case of someone entering my life and leaving again with no further contact.

He was replaced by Mr Thrift, whose teaching methods I remember much more about, he was in his thirties as far as I remember, and amused me by having a little oddity that fitted well with his name. Most teachers at that time would give a gold star for good work, these being made of gummed paper licked and stuck on the page, Mr Thrift however had an ink pad and rubber stamp and would give a red star, by these means saving the money which would have been spent on stars.

The only one of the three teachers I played up, by refusing to do something or other, very sensibly he refused to argue, picked up his books, told Mum he was leaving and the reason why, and told me he'd see me next time when he hoped I'd decide to be more co-operative. I had got myself into a position where, as usual I felt it impossible to back down but would have given anything to be able to take back my grumpy refusal to work. Next time he came all he said was are you now ready to work, the answer was yes and I never got myself into such difficulties again. Mr Thrift left on a peripatetic teacher being appointed for all the children who needed home tuition.

Eileen Alcock carried on from where the previous two had left off but the curriculum was much augmented and she would tell me how the other children she taught were doing and what they were working on, it felt like being part of a proper class, with an identity centred on Miss Alcock. At Christmas she would collect us all by car and take us to her parents' house, where a Christmas party had been arranged by her and her mother, splendid parties that provided the opportunity to meet her other pupils and ignite friendships that, in at least one case, lasted a lifetime.

English was always keenly taught and I recall her getting me to draw a border of lovely flowers and then draw in ugly sprawling weeds, and that border, she told me, was my speech or written work and the weeds were words that spoiled the whole thing, the only word I recall now is 'aint', but there were several other equally vulgar, but never curses, at least in the sentences of mine she heard or read. She would introduce a weed or two of her own, if we decide to call wild flowers, weeds, once it was a sprig of Scarlet Pimpernel she'd picked just up the road on her way from Alan Smith's house to mine, and once a Robin's Pincushion.

I remember how I hated the times tables, and how I memorised them one by one and then forgot them again one by one and how difficult I found reading the clock, I somehow missed the concept, or misunderstood the concept and dealt with it in the same manner as the awful times tables, I memorised the clock faces as presented and within a few days forgot them. Apart from these things my arithmetic was quite good and I only lost ground, until my ignorance of mathematics became almost total, when I went on to secondary school

Irene Alcock advanced my reading by loaning me adventure books, a series of books about a family of boys who were shipwrecked etc. and then a book titled How the Indians Got the Horse, which was the gist of the title anyway although I can't vouch for its accuracy. This book I loved as I had been interested in Native American culture even before Corley when Syd made me headdresses out of chicken feathers, the puzzling thing about my reading of this book was that I kept on getting one word wrong when reading aloud.

Chapter 31

Thong I repeatedly misread as throng. This became a terrific irritation as it seemed impossible to get it wrong only a few sentences, even a few words, since I'd been corrected previously. This was almost a Spoonerism in that I knew the word was thong but even so I would say throng, the same thing happened in the next book, The Children Of The New Forest, for the life of me I could never get Phoebe right, even when I'd been instructed in the pronunciation of what even now seems to me to be a deliberately clumsy word to read given the spelling. Frustrated, I blundered through the reading of the name over and over again and had to stop each time and tell myself to ignore the o. Other books followed, Treasure Island impressed me the most, and this I had finished by the time Miss Alcock came again, a book I could not put down.

One of the most interesting times was when we constructed a settlement of round huts utilising a modelling clay base with matchsticks interwoven with raffia for the walls a flattened cone with raffia strips for the roof. We also made racks for drying hay, again raffia. The whole thing may seem trivial to mention but it had all the aspects of life that fascinated me then and fascinate me still and show how attuned to my interests she made the lessons.

Just before the parting of the ways we started a project concerning leather and rubber, perhaps something to do with shoe manufacture, but in all honesty that's a guess based on the idea that Miss Alcock may have known that my maternal grandfather had been in the boot and shoe trade. We sent off to an organisation having to do with leather and back came a hard-back book full of information on tanning and preparing leather and a whole lot of information on rubber producing and manufacture into goods, this had samples of various types of rubber and a small vial of latex.

The project came to an abrupt end when I was ordered to spend the rest of my educational years at Baginton Fields School, the reason for the change was that Parry-Williams and his team had noticed a change in my character and decided I was becoming introverted, nothing wrong with introversion as far as I'm concerned it's just one of the avenues open to an individual to develop his approach to the world and in any case it was a bit late to try to change my way of being at ten years old. The truth is that I had indeed lost a lot of my outgoing and spontaneous ways because of the way Paybody and life in general had treated me, I had developed a deep distrust of anyone who might have an input into my life and found avoidance of such people and authority in general a better course of action than to engage with them, knowing that they would impose whatever they wanted, whatever I said, and all I had to do was develop strategies that would allow me to outlast their intentions.

I didn't want to go to Baginton Fields but Irene Alcock assured me that I would learn a lot more than if I remained her pupil, I wanted to believe her but later found out just how wrong even someone you do trust can be, however good the intentions.

My teddy bears had been my companions, the smaller of the two for as long as I could remember, being passed on to me by my cousin Bob when I was a baby, the larger, newer one Big Ted had a growl and had been bought for me as a replacement for Little Ted as he had lost most of his fur, his eyes were now sewn crosses of wool and the pads of his feet were replacements cut from my cousin John's school shorts after he had cruelly cut the originals off! But little Ted had a beautiful, caring and forgiving smile and I would just as well have died as swap him for any new friend. A great deal of my time was spent on my own recovering from bleeds or too ill to see anyone and my, now two, bears were very important companions to me. Came the day when Dad arrived home as I was playing a game where I was rescuing them from the snowy north, pulling them along in my upturned footstool equipped with a string harness, yes folks I was a team of sled-dogs. 'A boy of your age doesn't want to be playing with teddy bears.' says he, and clamps his lips into the line I knew meant trouble. I stopped my game and, almost in tears put away the Teds.

Then I started thinking about his words. I very quickly came to understand that he was talking nonsense, clearly

I was a boy of my age and equally obviously I wanted to play with the Teds otherwise I would not have done so. Looking for meaning behind the words spoken at me had become a reflex so I reasoned that what he meant was, I don't want you to be playing with Teddy bears, extrapolating I saw it was another case of 'Never let me catch you doing that again.' and resolved to play with the Teds only when his back was turned, and never to be caught! He was easily embarrassed and I realised later that his main concern was that no-one else should see me playing with the Teds.

Dad suddenly stopped going to the Devon after a dizzy spell on the top of scaffolding, when erecting ducting made by the firm convinced him that alcohol was the likely culprit and he decided to drop it altogether, or at least the traditional working-class habit of spending most of the time after work in a pub. That he could do so shows an admirable strength of character, later he would give up smoking in much the same way. The Devon gave me a lot of fun and also sorrows and I wasn't even wasting my time and money there!

Now of course, I see from so many other indications that he was a very self-conscious man, very easily embarrassed where other men would have taken things in their stride, still, at times it seemed as if Dad was reluctant to acknowledge my existence and that Mum was right.

His self-conscious fears must have been hard for him to manage but for me, at times, they caused similar distress to being ignored at the Devonshire Arms, the most excruciating of these was the time when, after a knee bleed I had to use the wheelchair and we were due to go out in the car, usually we would embark away from prying eyes in the back entry but for some reason me and the wheelchair were loaded aboard outside the front of the house. Dad got more and more agitated as, typically, he sat with his hands trembling on the steering-wheel, shiftily looking from left to right while Mum struggled to help me into the car and then stow the wheelchair. Suddenly he burst out with 'Can't you hurry up and stop making a poppy-show? We won't be doing this again!' I tried not to show my distress at being a poppy-show and I think I succeeded, but he needn't have worried I would not have allowed it a second time.

Much time was spent in clinics and the boredom of sitting waiting for my name to be called, was alleviated by hearing the way they would mangle Haughton as they called me for my turn. Parry-Williams' clinic was not so bad, after all I might meet a friend there, only spoiled when a trip to the Path. Lab. for blood tests was mentioned, until the arrival of a new SHO Dr Godiley.

I had, on the way to the clinic, become aware of an incipient elbow bleed and when Godiley asked me how I was I told him about the bleed that was starting, he examined my elbow from the other side of his desk, Mum and myself sitting together opposite, then suddenly dragged me half-way over the desk by my arm and told me that there was nothing wrong with it and that I was just playing my mother up. I yelped and cradled the arm, although there was nothing to see from his point of view the elbow was already a little painful and the joint felt 'sticky' which is not a term I can easily explain but invariably warned of a bleed. Mum also gave a yelp and stood up telling him he was cruel, cruel. The commotion alerted Harry Parry who strode over and asked what on earth was going on, then took Mum and me into another room and asked us to explain what had happened, asked us to wait while he had a word with Dr Godiley. A few minutes later back he came and told us that neither I nor any other of his patients would be seeing the misnamed Godiley again as he had been sent away and told he was not suitable to work with children.

Mr Bizzaro's clinic was wearisome, worrying and embarrassing, as there always seemed to be another horribly dispiriting plaster-cast, caliper or other instrument of torture to be offered or ordered, and invariably a shameful walk to be endured.

The clinic was held in a large gym- like room, a doorway at one end and much glass at the other, down both sides were cubicles fronted by curtains with strips of carpet running between opposite cubicles, and on arrival from the waiting room once the curtains were closed the order came to strip off every item of clothing and footwear.

Chapter 32

When Old Egghead arrived with his entourage of hangers-on one was required to walk across to the opposite cubicle and back while everyone watched for imperfections in locomotion. The nervousness and embarrassment was always there, both in the anticipation and possible humiliation, this did not happen every time but there was always a strong possibility. Being under the gaze of so many was an uncomfortable experience but given that the other surgeon Mr Penrose had his clinic on the same day, there was always the possibility that someone else would be perambulating up and down just a few cubicles away. This was a ritual humiliation made worse if the other paradee were a girl, some of whom were younger than me but some about to reach or at puberty and I would want to look but could never bring myself to do so because the watchers, including Mum would notice that too. Incidentally I had never felt ashamed of my skinny legs, until my father advised me not to worry as a champion boxer of former years had the nick-name 'Sparrow-legs', an illustration of how well-meaning advice often leads to self-consciousness. After his reassurance I dreaded every visit to that awful clinic of shame and humiliation.

On one of those visits I had a double punishment when on completing the walk I was made to repeat it, then Bizzaro announced that I was developing a problem with the arches of my feet and would be given cork inserts for my shoes on my next visit. Sure enough the inserts were ready for the next appointment and even more humiliation rapidly followed as this time I had to face the 'walk of shame' bodily naked but fetchingly adorned with socks and shoes.

Then off home with the inserts making me feel very unsteady on my feet, and after only a few yards I went over on my ankle, I knew of course that this could cause a bleed and my ankles had not been subjected to that as yet, through my care as to where I put my feet. I resolved to walk very carefully from then on and hoped that I and my feet would eventually get used to the inserts. I carefully got on to the bus and carefully alighted the bus with Mum eyeing me for bleeds as usual and walked up the street, crossed to the middle of the road when my ankle twisted more violently and I almost fell into the path of a car. Stumbling to the home side of the street I unlaced my shoes took out the inserts and threw them in the gutter telling Mum that was the end of the bloody things, put the shoes back on and angrily stumped back to our house. Mum didn't argue and even left the ridiculous, from my point of view, inserts in the gutter. Old Egghead's response must have been so muted on learning of my decision that I don't even remember it.

Clinic visits and hospital admissions around the issue of my haemophilia regularly intervened to ensure that I never felt settled. By now, visits to the dental department were also a regular feature; Mr Wood the dentist kept another gentleman in the corner of the room, who remained there as Mr Wood examined teeth and gums, this bearded man whose name escapes me was a sort of 'junior partner' or maybe an anaesthetist on tap but his habit of remaining obviously separate, fiddling with papers, smoking a pipe or watching from his corner gave an impression of a cross between Holmes' Dr Watson and a skulking Uriah Heep. Mr Wood on looming over and demanding access to the mouth would open his own, a reflex or perhaps a visual stimulus, so that while he inspected my teeth I could not only look up his nostrils but reciprocate the examination. I can report that while his teeth appeared to be fully present their appearance was awful, discoloured is polite but cannot conjure a picture of the mottled patches that decorated the interior of his maw, and his admonishment to keep up the brushing seemed to lack conviction, in my pre-Paybody days I would probably have responded with 'and you'. I had one or two cavities but nothing was ever attempted at that time apart from the application of silver nitrate. The efficacy of this I questioned at the time, as this happened once every three months and the cream bun I consumed afterwards, bought from the WVS run snack bar inside the hospital, was an instant negation.

These cream buns were the bribe or reward for attending the various clinics, the other treat was seeing one of the young women who worked with the clinical notes which at that time were returned by the patient on leaving the clinic and a new appointment made. There were several hatches in a wall and I insisted we always use the same one as the most beautiful woman in the world worked there, I marvelled at her appearance, always a sucker since virtually a baby for a pretty face and hers was the prettiest possible. I foolishly told this to Mum who next time told this vision of loveliness exactly what I had said, I was extremely embarrassed but she gave me such a sweet smile leaning out of the hatchway and if she could have reached I know she would have kissed me.

Nose bleeds were a big feature of my life at the time and I would often end up at Casualty where the offending nostril would be plugged and I'd have to sit in a cubicle on my own for what seemed like hours, why I don't recall, where was Mum, was I waiting for an ambulance to take me home, or was it a test to see if the bleeding would stop? There was a lovely nurse who was there every time, a novelty as most nurses I got to know and like were ephemeral presences, but perhaps the nose bleed phase was fairly short lived and this accounts for what feels now like permanence. This phase may have occurred when I was younger, or very soon after I came home from Corley because she would say let's find something to read, would go away and come back with several copies of a woman's magazine which had a comic strip series The Robin Family and she would read the words and we would talk about what the robins were doing, I look back with great affection on this nurse and her kindness, the delightful robins too, almost with tears. On one of these occasions the wait proved to be a very good idea as the bleeding switched to the other nostril and that had to be plugged as well. That day I went home with my mouth hanging open in order to breathe and for a few days I would wake up gasping and struggling for air as my mouth had closed during sleep, to counter this I slept on my back and let gravity hold my mouth wide open, a technique that worked but gave me a sore throat in the morning and a fear of flying insects in the bedroom so if a moth occurs I have to remove or kill it before I dare sleep. While lying asleep with my mouth open a large moth flew in, woke me and disintegrated in my mouth as I tried to remove it. Spitting and spluttering, trying not to breathe in the powdery wing scales whilst at another level knowing I was destroying it, in my panic, is something I've never recovered from. Even now I'm careful to keep my mouth closed and never lie on my back to sleep.

Other bleeds occurred regularly, keeping me constantly anticipating pain, sometimes excruciating at others just very bad. My technique if not sent into hospital was to take oral pethidine and read, read, read. Much against orders, medical and surgical, a hot water bottle would be applied; relieving the pain was all I cared about and to hell with the consequences. The pethedine was there next to the bed and I took it whenever it became necessary, having a short duration meant more often than advised. As the water bottle lost its heat I'd knock to let Mum know and she would refresh it, sometimes throughout the night, what a splendid mother! Sometimes this regime would have to be continued for forty-eight hours, I would see the sun go down, rise and go down again to rise once more reading all the time, and then as the pain died away I would sleep for hours and awake hungry, not starving but hungry after not eating for almost three days.

My biggest fear and something I took care not to let happen was running out of reading material. Aunt Flo, Mum's sister, lived in Hinckley and would come to see us 'On a nice day.' I would know which day when I awoke on that morning and would say 'Aunt Flo's coming today.' Mum would remind me that Flo had said a nice day not this one, but I just knew and before you run away with the idea that I only remember the times when I got it right I can only ask you to believe that this kind of thing happened to me all the time, if I said I knew, I knew! She shared a house with a companion, Edie Worthington who suffered badly from arthritis and who died some time during the 1950's. Edie left instructions that I be given her library of the complete works of Dickens, these volumes from Sketches by Boz through to Miscellaneous Papers proved invaluable and over the next few years I read each twice, including A Child's History of England. The first time I tried one of the novels I couldn't cope but the next year when I'd finally run out of alternatives I tried again and never stopped until I'd read them all. Reader's Digest also came in very handy and was usually left until the next bleed came along.

People would also send me books and magazines via my mother. One very disappointing parcel she brought in; she'd told me that Mr Brown had books for me and would sort them out if Mum went round for them, nothing happened until my next bleed when I was desperate for reading material Mum went and collected Mr Brown's offering which turned out not to be books but magazines, not that I totally despised them and indeed a few were quite old copies of Reader's Digest so readable at least and a change from the Farmer & Stock Breeder and The Smallholder, my usual magazines. I loved It 'Pays to Increase Your Word Power', still part of RD I'm told, and I remember the first time I got all of the questions right, not by chance but through knowledge and although I went on to answer every question correctly from then on the thrill was replaced by my usual fear of failure, putting me under intense self-induced pressure as a consequence.

The confusion over what was and what was not a book caused me constant irritation. There's a poem which has, and I probably misquote wildly, the line 'The kind of home where magazines are called books and books called rubbish.' this I found to be if not universal at least the norm among the people around me, the same people who 'didn't believe in psychology' and thought that the world they had their being in had never changed. Although I maintain that I was not a snob it's true that I spent a deal of time wincing and suppressing a sneer.

Chapter 33

My periodically overinflated ego was often judiciously pricked by the book I could never read; Penalties upon Opinion always got the better of me, being blisteringly dull, full of law suits, precedence and Judge's remarks going back centuries. This was one of the two books the household contained that were not mine and these were the spoils of Syd's grabbing of books from a bombed-out bookshop that had been dumped on The Dump during the war. Typical of Syd that one of the two books that fell to his share was practically unreadable in content, I expect his mates took the better examples. The other book however was very entertaining and I read it many times; Insect Ways on Summer Days told, in verse, the life and habits of various garden insects and had beautiful line drawings of each and was probably rejected by the local louts as poetry. It mustn't be assumed that my tastes were at all rarefied, I loved the Christmas annuals Dandy, Beano, Rupert and Roy Rogers, and in the summer came the Roy Rogers Album and I read many times the books from my early years. Every now and then a book written especially for children would come my way, two I remember in particular were Bim the story of a child with leprosy and his treatment in hospital and a book whose title could have been Andy Tinpockets who was certainly a character in the book. The annuals suffered a little by being required to take the place of a tray on which my passion for Plasticene modelling would be carried out. Modelling is not the correct word for my efforts were always three dimensional stories, with little men making camp fires, hunting, travelling in canoes and living in the wilds facing up to the odds. Sometimes characters and story lines from comics would be bent to my will, the central character always me, usually on my own and always ready to move on. Bucktooth The Boy Who Lived in a Barrel became Derek trundling the barrel along to new scenes as the old palled or people began to weigh heavily on his sense of freedom. Danny in his Iron Fish a kind of robotic metal, one-boy submarine rendered by me took me deep under the sea or porpoising along the surface facing adventure with courage and expertise. Other times a tiny Derek would take on and defeat Goliath, or camp out in a wild landscape complete with camp fire and skillet, canoeing down rapids, sleeping at night in caves always convenient to the river, or find a clearing with a water supply and build a log cabin, but always alone, making his own decisions and facing the consequences. The Plasticene was a constant source of pleasure as was reading, but ill in bed recovering from the latest bleed radio was my entertaining companion and educator.

The Morley's gave us a loud speaker which Dad connected to the Radio downstairs and brought into my bedroom, where the cable ran I have forgotten. The speaker was mounted on a piece of board and had an on/off switch and volume control and was just the innovation I needed, the drawback being that the radio had to be turned on downstairs before I could listen to my favourite programs. School broadcasts, Woman's Hour (very informative!) comedies, plays music and Children's Hour all livened up days spent in bed, a needed respite from reading as there comes a point where you can't remember anything in detail or general of the pages just read.

It is possible that the early years of some individual lives are for the most part happy, carefree and without the threat of immanent pain; perhaps this accounts for the fact that so many remember so little of their childhood and are inclined to scoff at those who do. My life, leaving out the time spent in the unfortunate Dotheboys Hospital, was relatively happy in spite of misunderstandings, physical pain and restricted opportunity. I was learning about the world from the radio, my extensive reading and home tuition and enjoying the process. The business of learning came to a virtual end with banishment to 'special' school.

Baginton Fields School for Physically Handicapped Children was never going to feel anything other than a punishment, an exile from a learning situation which I enjoyed and that suited my personality as it had in fact developed, rather than others wished it had, or hoped it might.

His insistence that I come off home tuition and attend special school is the only wrong decision I lay at Harry Parry-Williams door, although I understand the concern that I was becoming introverted, but the little boy who had shot him with a toy gun and told him he was dead and to lie down had gone into hiding. If Paybody had meant to cow me they had failed, I had merely become more cautious in all my dealings and the last vestiges of trust that remained I placed in one or two friends only.

Irene Alcock had assured me that I would learn more from school than she could teach me. I trusted her opinion and know that she genuinely believed this to be true. Though reluctant to make the change, I looked forward to the acquisition of more generalised knowledge but resented the dislocation from friendships and alliances acquired since my return from Corley.

Friendships at school were not exactly easy for me to pursue out of school, as most homes were without a phone at the time of which I write and the possibility of missing an arrangement due to a bleed was always there; if I said I would try to meet up it always sounded wishy-washy even to my ears. Anyway, because of the busing the whole set-up felt like being in hospital and as I've mentioned, but do not have a full explanation for, hospital friendships were mostly kept separate, sealed off from my home life and I found it troubling when the two became entwined. Loyalty and the search for continuity led me to feel, despite expecting to lose them, that I had friends at home already and one special friend so why should I seek new friends at school?

On my first day at the school another boy was given the task of showing me around, to protect his lack of innocence I'll call him Hugh Carpenter, he showed me various areas of the school and then ushered me into the assembly hall. This was in fact the end of the tour as Hugh judged it safe to skive there until the bell announced break and the end of his duty involving me. He was inclined to chat, asking me if I had a girlfriend, and then asked 'Have you seen Connie Barton's c - - t? Oooh it's all crinkly.' I'd only just arrived, was he offering to take me to see it as part of the school tour, being one of the sights (sites?) or was I to suppose his remark a prompt to test of my powers of observation with Connie Barton, genitalia on display, hiding somewhere in the gloom? Alas, I never did get a look, if only I had been a member of class3 I would certainly have had the opportunity, being part of a slightly higher sphere, class2 I missed the shows Connie and another girl put on for the boys. When I got to see her in the flesh she was a lovely looking girl even without a view of her famous vulva but I'll leave the subject of Connie for now. I have read that children with chronic illnesses or disabilities often have a precocious interest in sex, from personal experience and incomplete observation, I concur.

Life carried on just the same as ever except that school occupied a lot more of my day than home tuition had, and the busing to school was disruptive and not adequate to my needs at times. My friendships at home were put under pressure and I didn't care to make any at Baginton as already said, I was not unfriendly at first but soon learned to be, after the inevitable bleed saw me absent for a few days and things were stolen from my desk, at least this showed that the hooligans had noticed my absence. As bleed followed bleed and each time the teaching staff appeared neither to have noticed my absence nor to have made any preparation for my return, or to help me catch up once I had, I gave up on them as well and viewed them as time servers. Most of the boys at the school appalled me and the girls apart from stimulating my ever-deepening obsession with sex didn't interest me, I loved Denise.

Here's how my haemophilia was dealt with by the school: Forbidden metal-work, wood-work, gardening and cookery, I had extra periods of history and geography instead. Now isn't that curious? During those periods I could have been helped to catch up on the subjects I'd missed through hospitalisation and days off for bleeds, but no, huge gaps appeared in all subjects even the extra history and geography.

I arrived at Baginton competent in the maths I'd learned up to that point, started fractions, missed a little, went back to them, never finished them and the next time I returned the class were into decimals, this continued and sometimes I could put two and two together (pun intended) working back to the beginning from where the rest had reached but in very little time at all I was forced to give up on maths.

I did get involved in gardening once as arrangements had not been made to accommodate me, tut-tut such tardiness!

The gardening group had decided on growing vegetables to offer to their parents, this meant opening up grassland and making vegetable beds and anyone who knows a little about gardening understands that the first year wireworms are likely to devastate root crops and that potatoes are particularly likely to be heavily attacked.

The potatoes were ready to dig. I was stuck in a room and told to inspect the potatoes for wireworm holes as they were barrowed in, making a pile of the sound ones in one corner and the duds in another. Naturally I took my task very seriously, inspecting each tuber very carefully before consigning it to its designated pile, eventually a huge pile filled one corner, as the gardeners slaved to keep me well supplied with work, and a tiny sample of about five pounds in the other, the bell went for break and Mr Noonan and the diggers came in to view the harvest. 'Not bad eh sir.' says Tibbett indicating the mountain and then picks out a spud from the pitiful pile, inspects it and confronts me. 'There's nothing wrong with this one!' 'That's right, those are the one's without holes, other boys pounced on the wireworm ridden ones and demanded to know what was wrong with one specimen or another, if you looked carefully as it was possible to see that all of them had one or more holes. I had carried out my instructions to the letter as Mr Noonan knew. Any with a wireworm hole were to be discarded.

On one of my visits to my second home, the balcony on Sage Ward, who should come into the girl's ward to have her tonsils removed but Connie Barton, I was thrilled, was this my opportunity for a private viewing of her privates?

Chapter 34

In the event she did come to visit me on the balcony a couple of times until driven back by nurses, and both of those times we were very physically close in that she sat on the bed but the mephitic breath of one after tonsillectomy brought on nausea, as the smell was just the same as when I'd taken a blow to the throat and bled into my stomach vomiting up half-digested blood. How different life could have been but for an involuntary retch caused by a past bleed, Connie Barton, Connie even today your name provokes a frisson of desire.

Not long after this mixed experience of delightful closeness and disturbed olfactory another girl Maddy Drew rushed in, handed me a note and rushed out, the note read that she and another girl had, the previous night come on to the balcony when I was sleeping and 'did something to me'. What this was she didn't say, but asked for a reply which foolishly I gave her, telling her that if she came to the balcony again in the night I would reciprocate! Catastrophe, she immediately showed it to a member of staff and I was questioned about it. This was the last time I was admitted to Sage; from that point on it was always a side ward for boys off Cleaver, one of the men's wards.

When ill in bed at home various friends were allowed to come up and visit, who was admitted and who turned away seemed quite arbitrary, Mr Noise, the curate was always allowed entry, Al too and Elsie Roberts, but when Al and friends from school turned up one day, the party including a girl, they were all turned away, a shame because Alison lived quite near, was pretty, demure and sensible, and best of all I liked her.

It was the fashion for girls to wear lots of petticoats and a flared skirt at that time, and while I was recovering from a knee bleed Elsie came to see me dressed in all her finery. The only heating in the room was an old free-standing electric fire which was burning up the electricity at full tilt. We sat and talked, and after an hour Elsie rose to leave, turning at the door for a parting shot, skirt and petticoats swirled out and touched the fire, bursting into flames. She saw and her first reaction was to raise her hands to her mouth. I jumped out of bed, hopping on one leg. She backed away, giving out not screams but short yelps. I hopped after, yelling to stand still. I hopped she backed. A grab just before the flames got too hard to tackle and I gathered up the burning clothes twisted them together and squeezed. The fire was quenched. I barely made it back to the bed and fell on it, surprised that I had not sacrificed my hands, a couple of seconds more before grabbing and I would have. Elsie too was free of burns but again that was down to a few seconds, if she had backed away another step or so I would not have been able to reach her and just a little more would have seen her fall down the stairs. That's how close to disaster we came. Now she was worried about her parent' reaction to her ruined clothes but of course they were only happy that she was uninjured and grateful for my prompt action.

The Morleys had left and the house was sold to a family named Smith, I never asked so do not know if this was a coincidence, miracle or in some way manipulated but among the Smiths was Alan my distant friend from Irene Alcock's scattered pupils. Al had arrived, even better, he started at Baginton Fields, and so we caught the same bus to school and would meet at the start of the day sitting together as the bus took us on the familiar trip to nowhere.

The buses were in fact coaches that covered several routes across the city, picking up chronically sick and disabled kids as they went door-to-door. Home friendships were, as I'd feared, fading as a consequence of my being bused away while my old friends attended school locally. What seemed unremarkable at the time but odd with hindsight, is that my school friendships, I did eventually make some from among my own classmates, remained at school and my home friends now tended to be boys from Al's class: Gerald Houghton, Alf Smallman , Dave Martin, Philip Moore. Al and I would part at school and meet up back on the bus with the others always visiting us.

Each school bus or coach had a staff member on board to keep order and their instructions were that any child who couldn't clamber aboard unaided or with the assistance of family was to be left where they were. This gave me big problems as a knee or elbow bleed made getting aboard a real struggle, if the elbow was the problem then I had to use one arm to haul myself up the steps, putting strain on that arm and worrying that I might go through a day or so of having both arms compromised, and in the case of a knee Mum would have to assist as I took as little weight on the leg as possible. I have to say here that the bleeds had finished in these cases and it was just a question of being kind to the joint while it repaired itself.

After a while Mum was told that I had to go to school whether I had a bleed or not, this was partly my fault as I had started to insist that I was not going into hospital when I had a bleed, and so authority may have erroneously thought I was faking it so that I could stay at home, as no-one thought to ask me I can only speculate, whatever the reason my problems increased from there. Bleeds into joints are painful, I'm repeating myself but just in case we've lost that fact I re-iterate it, painful. So when the bleed was in progress I would refuse school, but as soon as I could cope with the residual pain Mum insisted that I go and if it were a knee bleed we would struggle to get me up the steps, moving from step to step by hauling with both arms while she gave me a boost behind. On reaching school I'd be told to get off the coach and would have to point out that this was impossible as, at the moment, I couldn't walk, at this point my struggle with my temper, which I was trying to curb would be very much stretched, and I would want to yell at them something like this: I'm here because you idiots have insisted, your shit-bag masters ordered it! But I won, and kept all vitriol to myself.

The first time they loaned me, for three days, a 'sleigh-ride', horrible contraptions made of wood on the premises, and were like a straight back chair with two small wheels at the rear, in fact quite useful for the more physically disabled and were customised to suit, their fault was that they were immovable unless tipped back onto the wheels which resembled castors or trolley wheels. Volunteers from among the less disabled kids would be assigned as pushers to each. When the joys of pusher and sleigh-ride came into my life it was humiliating and frustrating to have to wait for a specific person to push me wherever I wanted to go. As the regular user of the chair was off sick this 'pusher' had thought he was off duty for a while but now had me to contend with, in the circumstances he didn't tease me too much!

After that episode a manual wheelchair, and on one occasion an electric power chair, was loaned me, much better but always had me wondering on my way to school if one were available or not; I would have found the sleigh-ride impossible to go back to. The electric wheels were OK but not as good as a manually operated wheelchair. In fact my one go in the electric led to a monumental piling up of tables and chairs when I got the control jammed in 'forward' under a table.

By this time I had a circle of friends at the school and Bruce Household, who incidentally, at one time lived opposite Jim Cooper, asked me for my licence and when I gave it to him he endorsed it in the back. My licence was in fact my Green Card, with all the information on my medical condition, which from that day on I called my licence to carry on the trade, calling or profession of haemophiliac.

My first few terms at Baginton had been very difficult to get through, as I resented being sent there, and the promises about help when I needed it and a better, more rounded education were in fact mere reassurance, indeed there was nothing helpful in the 'must go to school whatever' policy and one day it came to a head when I got up in the morning feeling I might be starting an elbow bleed and by the time breakfast was over I was convinced but Mum insisted I go. By the second period I could stand the pain no longer and they sent me home in the school ambulance. This was bullying by authority which should not have happened, if they genuinely cared that I was losing out on education why not make efforts to help me catch up on what I'd missed,? There was plenty of time available in my school day. I suspect that my being there in accordance with acts educational was the important consideration!

The real shock was that authority didn't bother to help me catch up with the work I'd missed, they did nothing and on each subsequent occasion, sometimes on being admitted to hospital, they also did nothing

Chapter 35

Their incompetence stunned me and I have never fully trusted any professional again, knowing them all to be, at some level fraudulent. Maturity has revealed to me the truth that we're all fraudulent to an extent that's how the system works, but naiveté in the young is to be expected.

The fact that no attempt was made to help me is even more bizarre when banned from all subjects involving sharp edges, an overreaction as haemophiliacs, because of the inconvenience that a cut brings, are less likely to injure themselves around tools, being well used to taking care and anyway most small cuts are easily controlled by applied pressure. Extra history and geography, all well and good but surely this was an opportunity to help me catch up with, at least, maths and English, this would have been easily achieved if the teaching staff involved had been required to put aside materials to help me when I returned to school and I could have been found a quiet area to work on my own.

Oh those abysmal reading lessons, I suppose they were inserted into English classes as they had to be fitted into the curriculum somewhere, but shouldn't that have been remedial reading? Seemingly never ending, they dragged along at the pace of the slowest incompetent reader, and to follow on the page as the majority struggled with such difficult words as shed, soon and high, making a song and dance of caught or walking, nearly drove me into a screaming fit. I'd often get to the end of the passage and halfway through the next as the words drew me on and away from the stuttering, slow delivery of my fellow detainees.

It was these reading lessons that led to my nickname. I read fluently and quickly through a passage which contained the phrase 'He looked at them with an air of supercilious condescension.' and astonished, the mob yelled 'Does it really say that sir, make him read it again'. Sir and I complied and he asked if I knew what the words meant, while not being absolutely sure I gave an approximation drawn from the context and construction of the words, and he appeared satisfied. After that I was known as Prof and given a little grudging respect. Here are the questions begged: what was this lesson for, what did it teach, how was it broader based learning that would be better for me, and how did it benefit the barely literate members of the class, apart from applying a regular dose of humiliation? The same lack of reading skills remained the next week and the week after that, what a waste of time and effort, especially mine.

Before my professorship, I'd had no respect at all and, because I ignored the rest of my class as much as possible, was known as a snob, it wasn't snobbery but fear of becoming involved with boys who liked to hack and grovel in mock fighting, were largely uninterested in learning and endowed with a lack of wit causing them to mistake priggishness for snobbery. A prig I have to own to as their behaviour I found crude and repellent.

Then came the 'terrible' day when Mr Noonan spent a long time at the blackboard drawing a political map with all districts in different coloured chalk and the legend: The Union of South Africa in banner form. During break, someone changed the U to an O. The Onion, good! And astonishing as I hadn't thought any of them had the wit. Noonan was like a wild man pacing back and forth his face a high red smacked arse and his voice barely controlled. He asked for the perpetrator to own up and when no-one offered he told us that if this remained the case until the day's end the class would be kept in at every break and after lunch recess for a week.

After lunch that day I was assailed by a mob of classmates saying they knew I had done it and I had to own up, they'd misread my reluctance to involve myself in hacking and grovelling as cowardice and genuinely expected to be able to intimidate me into getting one of them off the hook. A lout named Gary Greatorex thrust his face into mine demanding I confess. Just attending the school was about as much as I could stand and as I was about to hit him as hard as I could, Spike Cosgrove who was with them said 'leave him' and they left me. Later Greatorex admitted that he had done it, what his punishment was I do not know having no interest in him or his friends, but later in the school year this Greatorex was suspended for some weeks after climbing up the huge stack of fuel which was surrounded on three sides by high brick walls and open at the front. I was there to watch him scramble up the coke with two members of staff floundering after him as their extra weight brought down more coke and he pelted them with it. A beautiful sight for which, belatedly, I thank him!

It was during this time that my friendships at school took off so that Spike Cosgrove, Bruce Household, Michael Redeson a fellow haemophiliac, and I became a group. Interestingly Spike was the only one I met for the first time at school, the other two I already knew. These friends made life at school a little more bearable although curiously my friends at school didn't include Al, we'd meet during the day but go our separate ways.

Mr Rees was now teaching science at Baginton and in the circumstances doing a fine job. The circumstances were these: We were not deemed worthy of being taught science so Mr Rees taught us without funding from the local authority, begging equipment from schools that were upgrading, or finding the cash from, I don't know where, his own pocket? I vividly remember the ancient science benches or tables set up for Bunsen burners, that he'd rescued from destruction when thrown out by another school, the Bunsens never followed requiring a gas supply, but the benches made the science room look the part at least and I would have enjoyed physics, chemistry and biology had they been taught, of course my steady decline in learning maths would have been a handicap, but even so. We did study biology one year but every other year of the downhill dash that was my school science career meant The Motor Car.

Because the school wasn't funded for science the science lesson was extra-curricular and at the start of the school year the class had a vote on what they wanted to be taught. The boys took the opportunity to have a block vote and this, all years except one, was for The Motor Car, by the third time of The Motor Car I hated the whole subject, but could have told you the workings of the differential gearbox, the internal combustion engine and several other things that were vaguely interesting but didn't grab my imagination. The year we had biology instead was a wonderful one and I learned things I hadn't known before, isn't that called education? I left school without formal qualifications and a tendency to swing between unalloyed belief in the capacity of my brain for learning and the feeling that if my potential had not been noticed then perhaps I never had any in the first place. My interest in biology has never faltered and in later years, by my own efforts with no concessions asked or given, I gained an A at O-level in Human Biology. I'm grateful that the vote went to biology that one year, lucky too, it was only because a couple of the boys had girlfriends, or would have liked to have girlfriends from the ladies of the class, and sided with the girls who always voted for biology and with a couple of rebel votes, including mine, that biology won the day. I know Mr Rees would have liked to teach physics or chemistry, and I would have liked to study the subjects, but these never got a look in.

The head, Mr Bulstrode often repeated in assembly how lucky we were to be taught by staff who could easily have got better paid, higher status jobs elsewhere but were dedicated to teaching children who might not have had the chance of any kind of education had it not been for Baginton Fields School, because there had been no provision at all for secondary school education for the likes of us in the past, so we were lucky indeed. I suppose it true that half-a-loaf is better than none to one starving, but I feel a few crumbs are nothing less than an insult. This was followed on one, or perhaps two, occasions with the announcement that Mr Rees was coming back to school on Monday and that he had suffered a nervous breakdown, what a wonderful teacher he was, and his efforts on our behalf took their toll on his health and with no science grant he had to beg, borrow and steal, to be able to teach us science at all.

This speech appalled me, I thought as head Bulstrode should not have settled for a part school grant but contacted the parents of the kids and asked for their support to ensure a full education for their children, in retrospect I see that he chose to believe what he said to us, the human capacity for fraud providing ample fuel for professional and personal self-deception.

Sometime during my early efforts to learn, it was realised by me and the staff that my eyesight wasn't up to scratch and I had to be fitted with spectacles, up to this point of revelation I'd imagined that the kids who shouted from a couple of hundred yards away only recognised me in a general sort of way and were calling to see if I reacted, after all I couldn't tell who they were so they must have been using some sort of trick, just as they did when pointing to a bird in a tree and naming it when all I could see was a fuzzy outline of a thing that may or may not have been a bird. I became aware of my short-sightedness when in class I failed to see what was on the board and everyone else could, this was mostly in maths. Two problems with my eyes, myopia and astigmatism were revealed by the optician and corrective lenses prescribed.

Chapter 36

The dramatic improvement in vision astonished me, and the realisation of how much I'd missed simply through faulty sight distressed me, however it explained a couple of things, how on a picnic with parents and cousins we played a version of cricket, and although given little dolly catches I never caught one, and on another picnic Dad discovered a hedge bottom nest with chicks which, despite his urgings and instructions that it was right in front of me, I failed to see, I confess now that he is long gone that in the end to placate him I put up a pretence of seeing that which he was determined to make me see!

Dad once again tried to bolster my ego by asking what they called me now at school, and told me not to worry if they called me 'winkle' or 'four eyes', once again I had not even considered that I might be teased until he mentioned it. Name calling had no effect on me, if one chooses not to react the gormless sods soon give it up and in fact no-one ever mentioned my specs.

My sporadic attendance at school continued to give me problems when chunks of subjects were just not available to me and still not one member of staff had the sense to see the problem and do something about it. Some subjects weren't so bad, music meant I had not been able to sing in class or listen to music, or had missed out on the position and what was expected of the percussionist in an orchestra, some of which could be inferred anyway. Art was problematic in another way in that the thing I was working on would disappear and I would be told to find it, the other bastards by which I mean my peers had hidden it under months of crappy efforts of their own. This did not bother me, as if I'd wanted to paint I would have done it at home, my ambition in the class was merely to remain inconspicuous until the next break time. I must have been good at this or Mr Corder or Stringwell, Cordwell or Stringer (one taught wood and metal work the other art, and string or cord being almost synonymous, memory cannot separate them with any certainty) would not have found it necessary to remark that I was 'like a chameleon'.

The school was required to stay behind after assembly, perhaps once a month, and Mrs Gray would get us all singing a hymn and then stroll along cocking an ear to those singing roughly in tune and anyone good enough she would jab a finger at and say 'you, choir' or 'you singing group' and when she got to me she would say 'you choir and singing group'. Alas, I used to ignore this, partly because I didn't know we had a choir or a singing group or where or when they congregated, partly because I despised the school and didn't want to get involved and partly because I might let Mrs Gray, the choir and the singing group down if I had a bleed at an inopportune moment. Not caring left me free, with a couple of mates, to sing alternative words to some of the hymns, such as Father, Son had Holy toast, suddenly Mrs Gray would stop conducting and say 'someone's singing the wrong words', a few someones were!

I resented being there but never took time off unnecessarily; my mother would not have allowed it to happen even if I had wanted to. I was in fact quite desperate not to be accused of using my medical condition for gain in any way, although sometimes people claimed I had, and because of the effort it took not to do so I would burn and seethe with indignation. It may well be that I took a few more chances with authority because I had no fear of physical punishment, but my chief delight was in achieving my nefarious aims without being caught.

Another mate, Gerry Northern, also from Al's class lived just a couple of streets away, and was corralled at Baginton because he had cerebral palsy, known to the multitude as spasticity, in other words he epitomised the archetypal 'spastic'. The natal brain injury that these individuals suffer varies in severity as does the consequent disability. I should say that Gerry came in the mid-range in that he could walk with an unsteady gait but with great stamina, I never once knew him to have to take a rest, and his speech while not perfect was understandable verging on normal, manual dexterity was imperfect and his head a little unsteady. Looking back on it he never introduced me to any of his other friends which leads me to the conclusion that he didn't have any.

Gerry would often pester me to kick a ball about with him, but mercifully his ball was lost and we could do this no more. It was an activity fraught with danger of a bleed, although I was very careful; holding back from situations where anyone else could just have put a foot in wasn't easy. Gerry announced that he had another ball and would bring it next day, sure enough he did. Dribbling a ball was an extreme task for Gerry with his unsteadiness and awkwardly dangerous to my ankles so imagine my horror when the ball he turned up with was a rugger ball, with which he proposed that we play soccer. I could see how embarrassing this was going to be and how the dangers would be multiplied. His certainty that it would be alright and the intriguing idea of giving it a go for its comic potential persuaded me and we kicked a ludicrous game on the gravelly edge of the tarmacadam playground, it was hilarious, not to say stupid and sure enough he stood on the ball and in falling grabbed hold of me. This was something he tended to do when his unsteady gait led to a trip or stagger and my tactic to, avoid injury to myself, was to fall down with him underneath to break my fall, so this I did, ending by sitting on his back, we both scrambled up and he told me 'that was your fault' then noticed that his thumb was bleeding and when he turned his hand over to look a piece of flesh opened into a flap and the blood gushed, he gave a scream and I told him to wrap his handkerchief round it and go to the nurse. He must have had stitches as it was a large wound, he always blamed me and we never played 'football' again.

The playground was a death trap when the partially sighted boys played their favourite game, these boys all seemed similar in build, looks and learning disability, and were victims I believe of a rubella induced syndrome in the womb, a guess that's all. Whatever the truth these great lumbering souls who all had massive feet, would link arms and charge around thus linked, great fun for them but terrifying for me as it was difficult to know which direction they would take, so I would stand with my back to the wall whenever they indulged their fetish, convinced that one day one of the little kids would be crushed underfoot leaving a spot forever greasy on the tarmac. With hindsight I suppose the ones with the better eyesight led the others and that it wasn't as random or reckless as it looked.

One of these, Roger Saint, rode the same school bus as I and would sit across the aisle from me, I tried not to stare but it was difficult not to as he suddenly screwed his face up into an even more grotesque look than normal and lifted up his hands to move his fingers about in front of his face, this, frankly, was funny to see but I knew better than to laugh. His temper was unpredictable. One day in the queue for the bus he turned suddenly and struck Connie Barton, who was standing quietly in line behind him, a heavy blow in the pit of the stomach, bringing her forward almost to her knees.

Some years later on Roger's last day at Baginton, as he was about to alight the bus for the last time, the lady who kept order asked him if he was going to say goodbye to everybody, he turned back and to my delight, spoke the best, short, summing up of life poem I'd ever heard and have never heard bettered.

I, I, I, I,.....Goodbye everybody!

I muttered goodbye back and a handful of the littlies from top-school piped 'goodbye Roger' and away he went. Apart from delight at the scene my other thought at the time was that the woman should have kept her mouth shut and let him leave with his dignity intact, no-one on that bus was going to regret his leaving and none were friends, sad but true.

My problems with missing days or weeks of school carried on although by now I was always able to borrow a wheelchair when necessary, some subjects remained very difficult, maths in particular, also, once Mr Liquorish had replaced Mrs Gray, music. But a happenstance unrelated to school had made it easy for me to keep up with subjects such as history and geography, ironic as I already had enough of these in school. My cousin John Sproul came to live with us for a few months on my Gran having to have her appendix removed. He finally went to live with his sister, and left his school books at our house, he was supposed to return them to school but said to me 'Fuck them, if they want them they can come and get them.' this they did not do and as the books were the same as those we had at Baginton I used them to keep up.

Music was much worse for me as it was now all theory and the writing of crochets and quavers on manuscript paper, needless to say I missed the beginning of this and came in at the point where everyone else knew how to draw and place clef, time signature etc. So, first lesson I'm able to attend, 'Right, draw your clef, two semi-quavers and' so on. I'm sorry Sir I don't know how to do that and I elicit the same old reply that dogged me throughout those years.

Chapter 37

'Yes you do, just get on with it.' It cost me a lot to own up to ignorance and this response always floored me and sparked me into solving the problems created in my own way, getting fairly close to the right answers in maths by breaking down the elements and placing the partial answers on an imaginary board in front of my mind doing the same with each element and then putting the separate answers together. With music I tried to copy the clef as I'd seen it and copied the quavers etc. from the boy next to me, not knowing of course what on earth any of it meant or how it related to music when I heard it.

Missed school work was recovered, supposedly, by the requirement to stay on for an extra year, what was meant to happen during the extra year I don't know, unless we were expected to suck in what had been denied us by scholarly osmosis from the educational aura that should have pervaded the school but didn't. It is my conviction that not all of the teaching staff were fooling themselves and their students into believing in the school, a bunch of my classmates confronted Mr Noonan when they said 'Sir, this is a school for dummies.' he leapt to the school's defence and told them the school was for physically handicapped pupils and those with what we would now call learning difficulties were not allowed into school, the kids challenged this by pointing out those who did indeed have such problems, and reluctant as I was to agree with the mob, I too could see that a number of people had intellectual difficulties as well as physical. Noonan reddened and said that Baginton Fields was a secondary modern school like any other secondary modern school, and I think he chose to believe it; unfortunately the differences were very apparent. I liked the man and had to decide whether his utterance was disingenuous or merely mistaken, at the time I chose to believe it to be the former.

So how was Baginton different to other secondary modern schools?

Top School was for infants and juniors but still Baginton Fields School.

We were bused from all over the city.

O-level exams were a rarity.

No punishment regime that included detention.

We were obliged to stay on for an extra year.

No end of year testing apart from statuary reading age and arithmetic age.

Hospital consultant's appointments held in school, during school time.

Physiotherapy applied in school, some kids taken out of lessons to attend.

No homework.

No science grant; that proportion of the school grant usually allocated for the teaching of science was withheld.

To repeat myself, I felt, after the first few weeks, that I was never going to get an education at the school; I felt that if I told anyone about my feelings only a bad result would follow and this I had learned at Paybody Hospital. If I couldn't sort things out on my own, then I had to outlast the situation with strength and cunning.

Hospital admissions continued throughout my time at Baginton Fields though now always spent in the boy's side ward on Cleaver.

I found Sue Lyons to be a wonderful Sister, running a ward efficient and cheerful. On a day I missed my lunch while down at X-ray, she offered to cook me potato cakes and scrambled egg, I liked the sound of potato cakes, having read of them, but the words scrambled egg brought to mind horrible hospital breakfasts, so I told her I didn't like scrambled egg, she replied that I would like them the done her way, so I agreed. I trusted Sue Lyons. Oh how delicious that meal, I can almost taste it now, both potato cakes and scrambled egg were revelatory; whenever I've tasted potato cakes since they don't compare and the scrambled egg was deep yellow, perfectly well seasoned, moist but not soggy. The stuff we were fed at breakfast was pale yellow, devoid of taste and swimming in water with globules of melted butter or margarine.

If you wonder why I don't compare my mother's scrambled egg, the answer is simple, when I got home I asked her for scrambled egg in the hope of repeating my joyous experience and she was non-plussed, repeating 'scrambled, scrambled, ooer whatever does he mean?' This I took as my cue to ask her for other things that I knew she would find exotic, something I'd read of, for instance 'A lightly coddled egg.' her puzzled assertion that I was making these things up was always mildly amusing.

I had come to dread the day when I would have to graduate to an adult ward as the small number of times I had been admitted to one or another men's ward until a bed became available on Sage had been awful. The men, invariably a miserable lot, complained, passed around grotesque newspapers devoid of news but heavily larded with the crassest of opinion and accomplished all to a soundtrack of what seemed to be competitive farting. The idea of a half-way house solution for pubescent and sexually interested pre-pubescent boys was a splendid one, and I shall always be grateful to the genius who formulated the plan.

The same old friendships and alliances built up and broke down every time I was admitted and discharged, and even now I feel sad that I could not bear to carry these friendship on once home again. Ray I remember with shame as he wrote me a letter from the ward, signed Ray, The Hawk in Hospital, and I never even bothered to reply, hoping he'd be there when I returned to the ward but he'd gone when next I was admitted. I kept the letter for many years.

Another event that saddens me is that I couldn't allow myself to prolong the contact with Julian who was admitted to the ward and had cerebral palsy, why he was admitted I don't recall but his CP was so bad his mobility was nil and when excited he flung his arms around and stiffened his body so that when sitting he would rear up alarmingly. I found his speech impossible to understand and yet I remember him as cheerful despite the nature of his disability, I would have perished from boredom in his position, not even able to turn the pages of a book.

The sad end to the story of Julian is that he came to Baginton Fields and was on my school bus every day, only to have me turn a blind eye to his efforts to get me to sit next to him. In the morning he was already on the bus and in the evening the ones who could not walk were loaded on first and the rest would form a line and climb on board when told, when I got on the bus, Julian would try to grab me straightening up in his seat and waving his arms about, I chose to ignore his invitation as his uncontrollable arm waving would have caused me problems eventually, that coupled with trying to understand his almost unintelligible speech over the buzz of conversation and engine noise would have been too tense an introduction to a day spent in an environment I felt neither happy nor comfortable in, and in the evening I preferred to unwind and forget the day's frustrations, still I regretted rejecting him. When Al started at Baginton it was easier as it was acknowledged that we always sat together but I could and should have at least smiled and nodded to Julian, alas I did not.

Paul, another boy who was virtually unable to articulate or co-ordinate movement, on my reading him a limerick about a young fellow named Paul and his abnormal tallness, would indicate to me to tell it again several times a day, once when his visitors were there, I would pause and he took delight in giving an approximation of his name in the appropriate place. His parents found it reassuring that he was neither ignored nor teased but brought into our company as much as possible and they thanked me for looking after him socially, embarrassing, as I found it hard to believe I'd made much of a difference.

Dante, son or grandson of the man who owned the ice-cream firm D. Di Mascio, was very slight and seemed too young for the ward, I can see his face in front of me now but remember nothing of our interaction. His parents were very complimentary to me for looking after him and Mr D. Mascio invited me to his ice-cream factory where I would always be welcome and could sample the ice-cream at any time. I never took up the offer. Di Mascio ice-cream was very well known in Coventry back then, the vans covering the city and perhaps beyond, in fact if children heard the van's chime they'd ask not if they could have an ice-cream but could they have a D. Di!

Cleaver Ward proved a lot of fun, my fear of being sent to an adult ward being allayed by the separate status of the boys side-ward, and we got up to some rare old tricks over the times I was corralled there. This ward too, had a balcony although no patient's bed was ever put out there. Remarkably though, a bed was occupied summer and winter by a non-patient. Charlie sold newspapers throughout the adult wards, ate in the staff canteen, and the balcony was his home. The end furthest away from the fire-escape and outside door, which was always open, was curtained off by an arrangement of old screens and equipped with an ancient hospital bed and equally ancient lockers, with most of his belongings in suitcases under the bed. We were told in no uncertain terms not to pry into Charlie's private space, as we would be in serious trouble if he caught us. With sparse white hair a drooping lower lip and a disabled arm which hung by his side, this brusque and forbidding individual inspired a sense of unease that guaranteed his privacy. How did this disabled non-patient come to live rent-free on the balcony?

Chapter 38

The Victorian hospital and the remaining buildings of Whitefriars monastery once comprised Coventry Workhouse and such a short time had passed since the infirmary had been renamed Gulson Road Hospital that my mother would tell me of her distress when one of my siblings was taken there and she cried, 'Oh no, not the workhouse!'.

Charlie had been a child of the workhouse and on its dissolution he didn't want to leave. Indeed there was no suitable alternative and he begged for, and was given, permission to stay, and the balcony of a men's ward was the obvious place for him, I suppose it was felt that with such basic accommodation he would eventually move on. This may indeed have been the case but I have no recollection of what happened to him during the time Cleaver was refurbished and the ward moved to Whitley and the boys, thereafter to Fennell ward.

I wonder if Charlie would be so compassionately treated today, I doubt it, a tidier solution to his accommodation needs would have been found away from the only home he'd known and not necessarily better for him.

Opportunity was always knocking on Cleaver and when workmen were carrying out some improvements they had to pass the window of the sluice and close to the balcony they were made uncomfortable by me and my team. The sluice was one of our favourites, due to the opportunity it provided to drench passers-by on Gulson Road; a sink, in front of a sash window, had a central nozzle that squirted water when a foot lever was operated, to rinse out the heavy glass urinals inverted over the spout. A judiciously placed thumb and a violent stab on the lever and the water could be directed across the grounds and onto the footpath, mostly missing our target but occasionally there would be a cry of protest when we would be back up the ward and reading in bed, just in case the victim noticed where the shower had originated. This stream we diverted onto the workmen, a much easier target as the water could be aimed straight instead of sideways; usually we hit the mark and considering how many times they were soaked their language as the water hit was most restrained, perhaps they thought it was the nurses' unique way of flirting!

Have you noticed how people have very little in the way of imagination when they bring gifts to patients, that horrible glucose drink, grapes or for some unknown reason, fresh free-range eggs and on the next visit are extremely concerned to know whether you enjoyed them? Any eggs that were brought into us did indeed get enjoyed while the workmen lasted, we would take them and while one kept watch the others would crouch near the balcony windows awaiting the signal that a workman was coming, then listen to his feet clumping along past the balcony and at my signal release the eggs, turn tail and get back to the side-ward, as we passed through the door we would hear a yell. Only when the workmen were gone would we go to the balcony to check the result, three dropped, three smashed on the ground, near misses, three dropped and only two on the ground one direct hit!

If Charlie saw you he'd make you leave, it can be imagined how irritating I found his attitude after all he was only there on sufferance and didn't own the whole balcony. Charlie once caught me and another haemophiliac, Brian Bidmead, riding up and down in the lift and sprang at us when the door opened on the ground floor, taking the lift back up to prevent our quick escape. We were both, supposedly, on bed-rest and certainly took a chance with the lift; we got to the stairs and felt relieved to get back to the side-ward without being spotted. This was not the warning it should have been and only a day later we were almost in more trouble.

A strange lad had come onto the ward, when I say strange I mean peculiar, he looked like a red-faced Billy Bunter and I suppose his behaviour would now saddle him with a diagnosis of Asperger's syndrome but in spite of his alien nature when next we commandeered the lift we took him with us, this was a mistake.

Brian pressed several buttons at once and in its confused state the lift stopped moving, while we waited for the lift to restart Brian took it into his head for no reason I could fathom, to explain to our companion what a woman was called 'down there' pointing to the loins of

Billy Bunter, it's spelled see, yu, en, tee says Brian, one of the few words he could spell, and don't tell anyone I told you. The lift finally decided to take us to our floor and Brian and I exited trying to sneak back into the ward but our companion rushed up into the main ward yelling at the top of his voice his new found word, with the nurses looking at him as though he had gone mad, 'Would you look at him now, what's the matter with the poor thing.' and louder 'Derek Haughton what have ye' done to him you bold boy'! Spelling being one of his weirdnesses and Brian spelling it out to him the nurses had been assailed by a Billy Bunter look-alike shouting sunt, sunt, sunt at them.

He was a maths wizard and could also draw really well but his social skills were nil and he had some very strange ideas about the comics that were brought in by his parents. The Beezer he insisted on calling the Buzzer, even after being required to spell it he insisted that b, e, e,z spelt buzz, and even stranger was his idea of a joke. In another comic, possibly The Lion, a character was called Robert the Robot his version was Robert the Robert and he claimed that robot was an alternative spelling of Robert and was a joke on the part of the writers of the comic strip.

Every bed had a set of headphones, a box on the wall giving choice of station and volume, a standard arrangement, and whenever I was on the ward, unmissable was the late shipping forecast and we all kept awake, headphones on, sitting straight up in bed waiting for the traditional 'Goodnight gentlemen, good sailing.' when we would salute and say 'Goodnight Sir.' and settle down, night nurses new to the ward would come running to see what we were so verbally united about, but we, my cohorts and I, were already snuggled down and apparently sleeping.

Even a well-run ward is subject to unfortunate circumstance from time to time. A particularly vivacious young nurse, persuaded to dance round the side-ward with one of the boys, found herself caught and sent to be disciplined by Matron. We saw the proceedings, as the windows overlooked matron's office and we saw the back of Matron at her desk with our happy little nurse facing while receiving a lengthy dressing down, we saw her wipe away tears and turn and leave the room. Later we heard two other nurses talking and saying that really she had been quite lucky to be given a short suspension but that Matron had promised one more breach of the rules would lead to her training coming to an end. I never saw this nurse again as the next time I was admitted she had moved on to another ward, but have always felt guilty as I should have warned her how unpopular she would be if caught cavorting.

A word here for old-fashioned Matrons, the Matron of Gulson Road Hospital Miss M. Donagh ran the wards with great skill, efficiency and a calm authority. She visited each patient daily, open to complaints or requests and on these ward visits every closed door would be opened and she would check that nothing was amiss, right down to the linen cupboard which had to be kept tidy. Any problems would be reported to Sister, and Sister would make sure that the matter was addressed, reprimanding any culprit. All the nurses knew that if Sister told you to do a thing, you did it, no demarcation between cleaners and nurses, spillages were attended to immediately. This is how it should be, if a cleaner is not available then a nurse should be assigned, as the patient, friends and family don't care who does the job as long as comfort and safety are paramount. No naming of hospitals, but I have seen, over recent years, spillages, including blood, used towels, soiled pyjama bottoms and bloody toilet seats ignored for hours, days and in one case a whole week.

As already said, even the best run hospitals lapse into inefficiency and I was once prepared for surgery, the whole thing as it was done at the time, my protests being ignored. So, dressed in a hospital gown, a green hat and big woollen socks I tried once more to persuade the nurse that I was not supposed to go for surgery that day.

I had been admitted with severe toothache and was due to be transferred to Birmingham General for a tooth extraction this being a risky business and Birmingham General having the haemophilia know-how and a brilliant dental department, but due to an administrative blunder the nurse had me on her list for prepping. The matter came to a head when she insisted I have the pre-med injection, always administered on the ward, and checked her list again, showed me I was on it and undermined my certainty enough to allow her to give me the jab, which, on the plus side provided the opportunity to experience a pre-med. Sleepy and with a dry mouth as warned I kept myself awake and waited for the SHO Dr Dent to pass the side-ward as he came on duty, I waved, he passed the doorway, skidded to a halt and stuck his head round the door with a horrified look and hared off up the ward shouting for Sister.

Chapter 39

I was asked why I'd let it happen and I protested I'd only complied when shown the list, and then I allowed myself to slip into a drugged sleep.

A more distressing incident occurred when the doctor given the task of setting up a plasma drip couldn't manage it and after a prolonged attack of arm sticking he decided to attempt a cut-down on a vein in the ankle, again this did not work and now, with the ankle vein bleeding onto the bed, he switched his attention back to the arms. How long the torture would have lasted I don't know but a doctor, I think named Darcy, who was almost good at the game of Draughts came along and washed his hands at the sink next to my bed, winked at me and said did the other doctor mind, in the meantime tightening the tourniquet, but he could usually find a vein just here and did so first time. I loved his style and of course was very grateful for the intervention.

Dr Darcy and I often had a game of Draughts together which I always won and he'd throw up his hands and saying 'He's done it again!' laugh and walk away shaking his head, one of the few doctors I admired and actually trusted, I hope I learned from him.

On Cleaver I received my one, and so far only, death threat. I was a member of the Anti-Fascist League and insisted on wearing my AFL badge everywhere, even on my pyjamas and this usually provoked right wing jerks to expose their true beliefs but this time it provoked more than pathetic ravings about anyone perceived as different and when I came back from an X-Ray under the pillow was a note reminding me that I was vulnerable in hospital and that it was likely that I would not wake up one morning unless I removed the badge and kept my mouth shut. I never reported the note and kept my badge on. I know it was one of the porters who put the note there, one of the two who had taken me down to X-Ray, perhaps you might think it a joke but I don't think so as if handed to Sister it would have led to an investigation and almost certainly, a dismissal.

I had joined the Anti-fascist League when introduced by another boy at school and wore the badge with pride and a hope to flush out the nationalistic bullies I suspected of running, in part, the school. Their outrage would have driven them to take away the badge if they, indeed, existed, again my arrogance prodding me into a ridiculous stunt. I knew there were traditionalist elements among the staff and remain certain that one at least deplored the harassment of the rank Colin Jordan who at that time still taught maths at another school in Coventry and whose fascist supporters regularly attended wrestling matches where they would be barracked and taunted by AFL members. Jordan himself was often subjected to similar treatment on leaving home or the school gates and I'm convinced that the embarrassment and pressure thus put on the local authority, added to his own inglorious antics, led to his dismissal from his teaching post.

The porters in general were a bad lot, the head porter known as the Baron and the porters lodge as his castle, a castle where at least one young nurse underwent sexual harassment by the Baron and his crew. I heard them boasting of it, and the inference was that more than harassment took place, the nurse was very young and I have reason to believe as sexually obsessed as I. Very young because she was what was known as a Cadet, and deserved to be treated better whether she appeared to encourage them or not.

This same Cadet had burst into a toilet compartment before I had the chance to lock the door saying 'Now's your chance.' it turned out to be another chance missed as it was altogether too much of a shock and anyway I was a couple of years younger than her and perched on the crapper. An insalutary grope or whatever she offered was not what I wanted and neither by word looks nor gesture had she shown any interest in me at all until rushing into the toilet, pushing the door to and standing with her back against it. I could, no doubt, with a little warning and if I hadn't been desperate to evacuate my bowels, have enjoyed whatever she proposed despite my reservations, contemplating the event later I thought I might behave differently next time it happened but it never did.

I utterly rejected the gormless racialist/ nationalist clap-trap which seemed to be spouted by most of the people around me especially among the patients; these barely conscious types would be very subdued after a black nurse had been obliged to administer a suppository, or look after their needs in any way and would often cry when they thought no-one was looking, occasionally yelling 'I don't want a black doctor' with the added drollery 'I fought in the war for this country'. My lip developed an almost permanent curl of contempt.

One of the more vociferous curs yelped his stupidity even down to not wanting toast if the 'black' had made it. He afforded me many a laugh and his subsequent fate a quiet smile and direct look. I went home with him in full flow but when I came back with another bleed, his appearance and demeanour had both suffered a severe change; though considerably more morose, he had nothing to say, especially concerning black or brown or any other colour of nurse's and doctor's complexion; his condition had worsened, his own complexion turning to mahogany and he looked into my eyes receiving the direct look and smile already mentioned. There was no need for more.

He became increasingly abject and even allowed himself to defecate where he stood, untroubled as the nurses scolded him for not asking for the commode. Poor chap I think he was in the end stage of whatever disease he suffered from and the next time I came onto the ward he was dead. The words, serve him right, I have to own, were what I thought at the time and, indeed, the irony had a beautiful symmetry, a black hater turning black.

A bed-making round was always one of the highlights of the morning and a chance to have a laugh and joke with the two nurses assigned to the job. It happened that my toe somehow got caught on one nurse's apron at crotch level and she said, seeming so droll at the time, 'Hang on there Breda, Derek's after toeing me.' and once again I was told I was a 'Bold boy'. It was clearly and emphatically an accident your honour. Every exam time the nurses would get serious with no time for joking around and on one occasion the talk was all gyny, I learned to recognise vaginal discharges linked to their respective conditions when others of my age didn't even know what the term vagina meant. In fact silly boys would often ask if you knew 'the proper name' for a girl's c - - t and say it was written on every penny and point out Regina, one poor specimen when asked why the Latin for that intriguing portion of a woman's anatomy should be on a coin replied 'because it's the Queen', an answer interesting for its lack of any meaning at all.

I very quickly learned to take my own teaspoon onto Cleaver, the men being served drinks first, by the time the trolley reached us teaspoons would have run out. I kept a small tin box permanently filled with objects likely to prove useful on my next admission; included with the teaspoon were the blade from a pencil sharpener, cotton and needle, string, lump of Plasticene, stubs of pencil, a pocket notebook, plasters in case of cuts (if I could deal with a cut myself, no need for tedious explanations of the origin and possible confiscations) a safety pin, a small cup-hook and most importantly analgesics for self-treatment. Pain relief could be almost non-existent in hospital, 'Doctor has written you up for a codeine.' codeine was what I took for headaches at home, aspirin being a bad idea for haemophiliacs and paracetamol not yet on the scene. I have no idea about the milligram situation, perhaps the codeine in hospital was 'stronger' but whether or not it didn't control the pain, to use a crude phrase of my father's it was like farting against thunder and after being left in agony a couple of times I took matters into my own hands.

Cleaver was moved to Whitley Hospital while the ward was re-furbished although we never actually got back to it as the ward staff and all appurtenances when returned to Gulson were now accommodated on the ground floor.

At Whitley the boys were accommodated on the men's ward as a group at the end closest to the entrance

Four individuals among the adult patients stand out in my memory, the amputee who had an artificial arm that was attached to a leather and metal shoulder brace. On the way to morning ablutions he'd walk up the ward minus his pyjama top swinging the artificial arm like a propeller by twitching his shoulder, the arm swinging round faster and faster with a whirring sound that eventually reached a high-pitched whine. I think that his example was a good one; here was somebody who not only chose not to hide his disability but to convert it into fun for the entertainment of self and others.

A young man unable to get out of bed, or even sit up and had the dreaded cot-sides fitted to his bed, told us that his problem was epilepsy and indeed he had a couple of seizures while on the ward. Epilepsy had struck without warning and had worsened to the point we saw now in only a matter of months, he'd been perfectly fit until he reached twenty years and then in his words, the epilepsy took over. All his front teeth were missing, knocked out, from falls when seizures struck, I still have that image of him struggling to communicate with us through very slurred speech and know that a lot of his difficulties were caused by the drugs used to control the epilepsy. Sadly, no name is associated with the image but it remains a powerful reminder of the randomness with which illness may strike.

Mr Singh was on the ward twice when I was admitted, and would ask my advice about English pronunciation and about words that were not to be found in his language books, 'How you say this, Derek?' or, pointing, 'what you call that?' Some things he saved up to ask me, as he knew I would not be upset or laugh, 'Derek, what you call these?' Jouncing imaginary breasts in front of his chest, this was one that needed thinking about, so I explained the importance of knowing when to call them breasts, mammary glands, or tits.

Chapter 40

We had a lengthy discussion about the matter and I wished I'd left mammary glands out, also the impolite tits and the like, when I just couldn't get it through to him that in everyday conversation mammary glands would make him seem like a nut-case and knockers unnecessarily coarse. The last time I saw the man he asked what had happened to my friend John, since I had no friend John and any names I threw at him he denied, 'No, no your best friend John.' this part of the conversation petered out although I still feel puzzled by the John character. He then told me 'you common mistake' and when I asked what mistake he pointed to my upper lip and repeated 'you common mistake'. Then I did have to acknowledge my mistake, what he'd said was 'You coming moustache.' the latter word not being one he'd asked me how to pronounce it sounded like mistake. When I acknowledged the fact, he asked if I had a girlprend, I considered Denise my girlfriend and told him yes. 'You tell girlprend I have plenty money.' he eagerly told me and I wondered just what he meant by girlprend. Not one of the other patients spoke to him being victims of the low-level racism club that fears to be seen talking to an outsider; rabid Nazis are never a danger, but the salt-of-the-earth, easily led, ignorant types grease the wheels of the fascist juggernaut, potential bystanders or worse at every atrocity.

A man who convinced me of the horror of sticking to one thing all your life was an old printer who worked for the local rag. He may have been retired but I believe he was just about to when struck down with illness and confined to one of the giant cots, not a bed with cot sides' added but the sort that only needs a barred roof to be fully cage-like. He would sit every day, at the foot of the cot with his legs through the bars fiddling with controls and levers that only he could see and was known as 'pop', with his snow-white, receding hair it wasn't hard to see why, often his hospital gown would be concealing nothing and the nurses would say to him 'Come on pop, cover yourself there's ladies present'. Who the nurses were to him is a mystery, but he often told them 'All I need is Carter's Little Liver Pills, they don't listen but that's all, Carter's Little Liver Pills.' He thought that me and Brian Bidmead were apprentice printers and would tell all who bothered to listen that he didn't like the new apprentices because they were much too cheeky and that he'd have to report us if we didn't shape up. Bidmead used to tease him about the Little Liver Pills, but I don't remember teasing him at all.

I do regret teasing and I suppose it must be called bullying a schoolmate who came in for reasons of what we might now call respite, his parents having gone on holiday for a week, for the first time in years; no doubt his admission was at the insistence of Harry Parry Williams, whose compassion could overrule any protocol. That's how hospitals were, and should still be, run. Anyway, this lad suffered from muscular dystrophy and was unable to move more than his head and arms to an extent, but had no strength to fight us off, we shoved some grapes down his back and Bidmead patted him and squashed them, he gave a grimace and seemed to be taking it in good part, but I was hit with the realisation that he could do nothing else and what we were doing was bullying someone virtually defenceless. I stopped and managed to distract Bidmead from the sport and the rest of our schoolmate's stay was uneventful. Writing this has been hard, I'm still ashamed of my part in it, but realise it was more sad than cruel, and was partly a case of having nothing physical to do and grasping any opportunity to vary the monotony, in the unlikely event that anyone remotely connected to this outrage is reading this, I apologise.

Brian Bidmead had never been a friend of mine, either at school, where our paths seldom crossed, or in hospital on the several occasions we were in at the same time, it was more a case of being thrust together by circumstance and the understanding of what it was like to be a haemophiliac, and it was good to see a familiar face so we formed a gang of two. At the age of thirteen most boys are showing an interest in sex and we were no exception, stealthy masturbation being our thing, both confined to separate beds let me add and both unaware how obvious we were being. I didn't like Bidmead or his attitude, his crude and aggressive nature or anything about him but we'd spent time in hospital together so often I could empathise and anyway I felt sorry for his mother.

After a time the staff decided our friendship, as they chose to think of it, was unhealthy and we had to be separated. The first 'cure' that was tried was to move me to the opposite side of the ward and then the prescription was torn up by letting him come across to me in a wheelchair, he tried to scramble onto the bed, but I made it difficult and he fell to the floor, hitting his elbow and causing a bleed, immediately I blamed myself and felt very sorry for him as the pain got worse, though at its worst it didn't last as long as my bleeds did. For some reason they moved me back beside him and at the same time decided to see if religion could help by asking the visiting C. of E. vicar, Rev. Lumpton, to give us some instruction in the faith. On his next visit he told us it was time to begin Confirmation Classes and we must make a start next day.

A cluttered dayroom, never used as such, more a repository of 'could be usefuls' saw us in wheelchairs awaiting the Rev. who soon joined us wearing a bicycle clip on one leg, 'Well boys.' says he, 'Let's make a start.' and proceeds to talk sex. 'Now, when a man and a woman are very fond of each other and marry, on the wedding night they kiss and, and.....er...I think we'll carry on next week.' As he got more into this very brief speech so his excitement grew and his legs jumped up to his chest, one at a time in a distracted rhythm. I don't suggest that the speech as rendered by me is in any way verbatim and the length of the instruction was a little more prolonged, around ten minutes, but the gist is true and there was an awful lot of repetition and increasing excitement, he seemed reluctant to leave his seat and told us we could go, as we passed out of the door Bidmead said 'There's something wrong with him!'. A week later we witnessed exactly the same performance and after that the 'confirmation classes' were dropped by mutual consent. A couple of years later my cousin and several of her friends took 'confirmation classes' and she told me that the vicar was sex mad, as all he talked about every time was what a man and a woman did together when fully licensed. She called him Lumpy and my suspicions aroused I asked his name, Reverend Lumpton she replied and I told her he was only up to his old tricks, fortunately all the girls thought his antics funny, with the legs jerking about and the stuttering and starting, and he never progressed to anything more overt so I took no action.

Bidmead told me that he had had sex with his sister, this did not shock me, I had no sister but could see that proximity might have stimulated them both into a bout of exploration and experiment, although I found it unlikely that any girl would have been keen to be futtocked by him, anyway this was probably a bragging exercise, his general crudity seeing no reason to leave his sister out of it.

One last attempt at a cure of my perceived 'attraction' to Bidmead involved a young nurse possibly seventeen, who ostensibly gave me a bed-bath which went on for over an hour, with Bidmead demanding to know what was going on behind the screens. After the bed-bath we talked and talked and got on very well together. Bidmead tried to suggest the episode had been crudely sexual. I did wonder if it was some kind of test, but didn't care as I was very attracted to her. Next day she gave me a book to read, A Kiss before Dying by Ira Levin, I never saw Bidmead open a book and he never gave me peace to read, so this had to wait until I was home again. Living Doll by Cliff Richard (Cliff Richards at the time) was no. 1 in the pop charts so I must have been fourteen and it was just as well that the nurse and I never got any closer or we might have both been in trouble! We never got the chance, and how I regretted it as Old Egghead re-entered my life.

Parry Williams decided that the best thing was to separate my companion and I by transferring Bidmead to Dotheboys, Hospital and when Bizzaro came he decided to take us both, the pair of us had a knee that refused to get back to doing a knee's job and so orthopaedic treatment was necessary, Bidmead's being worse than mine. On the day we were transferred my nurse friend cried and I did nothing but look and feel distressed........

It was back to hell for me, although Bidmead soon adjusted. So it was traction for both of us and it only took a little while until my knee decided to behave itself and then it was physiotherapy until I could walk unaided around the ward. Before that happy day one or two things happened; I had never joined the scouts as my Dad and Grandad said all it was good for was making cannon fodder but the ward had its own troop and invited to join I gave it a go. I lasted a week. We had the tray full of objects game, where the tray is covered by a cloth which is whipped off and you try to memorise what's revealed, then the tray covered again. I was doing well when Bidmead who was doing badly asked me to tell him what I could remember, I helped by telling him one thing and never got a chance to tell him more as the scout mistress pounced on me, called me a cheat and threw me out of the group, Bidmead stayed, this was no surprise, it seemed just the way it used to be when I was so much younger.

We were taken to a room for bathing once a week and helped onto a scrubbed wooden table to be washed, a young male nurse was detailed to wash me and when it came to the genitals he handed me a flannel for the job, contorted his face, thrust it into mine and snarled 'You filthy little devil.'

Chapter 41

I had no idea at the time why he should say this as he'd asked me to wash myself and how was this to be accomplished if not with flannel and hand? I had no idea that I had been labelled 'queer', it didn't occur to me as all my sexual instincts and longings were focussed on the opposite sex, one girl still my obsession and the focus of my fear.

I noted that the same old ragging and teasing remained a feature of Paybody and managed to keep myself away from harm, if you leave out the previous two incidents, but I worked hard at getting out of the place just in case I inadvertently brought myself into focus. Another boy, however, was the recipient of the staff's contempt and verbal bullying. This lad who was on the large size had, I suppose, a problem with his back and was encased in plaster from hip to neck. Built into the front of the cast was what looked like a medieval torture instrument as it could be adjusted every few days by giving half a turn with a spanner to gradually straighten the posture. So many of these things looked like instruments of torture, it made you think! The cast stopped this boy from sitting, he could lie down, walk around or kneel, so to read or eat he chose to kneel next to his bed. The oft repeated cry would be 'There goes the bishop again, always saying his prayers.' Perhaps amusing heard once but in his position it soon got very wearisome as this comment would emerge each time he was forced to kneel. Eventually he took action by going along with it and wrote a letter to the Bishop of Coventry asking how one went about becoming a bishop. To his credit the Bishop replied and explained the hard work and commitment needed, the poor boy showed the reply to a member of staff. If he had asked my advice I would have told him no, don't, things will only be worse for you but he didn't ask my advice. Sure enough a hue and cry was raised as the letter was passed around, and the general comment was what an idiot, he thought you could become a bishop just like that, how stupid can you get or words of that kind. Poor kid, tears and his head hung down, he'd tried to take it all in good part but hadn't understood that the people he was dealing with were of the lowest sort. He stopped talking and looked whipped for the few days longer I was there as the yapping and name calling dragged on and on.

Just a day before I left for home a younger boy who lived over his father's bicycle shop just down the road from my home came in with a broken leg, I knew John Wareham but we were not mates as he was, as I say, younger than me. I shall always now be ashamed of rejecting his appeal for help. He was desperate to relieve his bowels, and I had heard him ask for a bedpan on two occasions and be told he would have to wait and a bedpan round had been done an hour ago anyway. He called me over to him and begged me to make them get him a bedpan as he couldn't hold on much longer. I told him no, and that was a harsh thing to do, but my involvement would have made matters worse for him in the long run and would have caused me to be spot-lit for the next few hours until I left. He asked the staff again in distressed tones and was ignored, the next thing I knew he was crying and lying in a soiled bed. Then they came to him, 'This little boy thinks it's alright to go to the toilet in his bed, he couldn't be bothered to wait a few minutes.' I left next day thankfully as I would have been in trouble myself because I would not have been able to listen as his dreadful deed was harped on about day after day, especially considering the guilt I felt.

I was free forever from the Paybody experience and Bidmead too, although the latter accosted me when he came back to school telling me to look how well he was walking and that I was bent forward 'Look at me compared to you, you should have stayed.' He was indeed walking better than me but this was fine, my imperative was to get out of that place.

At home my inner turmoil went on, I was desperate for Denise but so frightened of getting hurt, especially if we had established a sexual relationship as I knew that would make me even more terrified of losing her. This had the predictable consequence of elevating her to an untouchable position, the one I wanted in every way, but the one I had to keep away from in my, for instance, masturbatory fantasies. Remember that I never had any sex education and tended to make it up as I went along, the only thing my father did was to procure from somewhere a book which he told me he'd read at my age, this in itself was a revelation as the only book I'd known him to read, and even that that he never finished, was about Japanese atrocities in world war two. The book he gave me, written by Dean Farrar was Eric or Little by Little, and concerned the gradual degradation of a public school boy who eventually loses everything. I remember little of the story but an injunction on Eric to remain pure. I took the book at the time to be a treatise in novel form on the lowering effect of masturbation and resolved to stop the practice as soon as the idea had been satisfied this time. Sadly, practise made perfect and I quickly decided to ignore my father's advice if indeed, he had been trying to advise me. He was much too late anyway I'd been shown the trick by an older boy, who does not feature here, years back when I could have all the feeling and none of the mess, in fact I was shocked on the first occasion semen was produced.

Dad remained a fascinating study and still took delight in informing me that I would never have to look for a job as I would be accommodated at Red Lane where the family business had relocated.

I had got my hands on a plastic replica of a German Luger pistol into which one loaded ten, two centimetre long, plastic 'bullets', I must emphasise that this was a toy, not a model and not full size, but very accurate over about twenty feet and if bare skin was struck, quite painful. Dad was sitting at the table reading the newspaper and from my position by the door I wondered if I could hit a bottle on the table in front of him, knowing that the ping would startle him, he'd look round and see me and give a chuckle. The shot was accurate the plastic 'bullet' hit its target, the ping was satisfactorily loud but the ricochet took it smack onto Dad's forehead right between the eyes, no chuckle from him, he rubbed his forehead, gave me a little look over his diamantes, muttered bloody hell and went back to his paper. We were both very fortunate that it was his forehead that bore the brunt of my target practice, and that his reading glasses remained unharmed.

I think he accepted it as just another example of his bad luck. This is a theme I know quite well, as he often says that he is the picture of bad luck, and with the benefit of hindsight I am convinced that he actually suffered from a mild form of seasonal affective disorder as he always said he dreaded the winter and hated autumn flowering plants as they reminded him that winter was coming, he seemed resigned to the winter months producing catastrophe.

Disturbing news concerning The Dump appeared in the local paper, plans were afoot to build on it, this incensed the various gangs who considered it their stamping ground, already a great deal of The Cornfield had disappeared and been incorporated into the grounds of Lyng Hall school but we still had The Dump and another field of open land out to Wyken Parish Church and church hill. My Mum and Dad grumbled a bit and said when they moved in they and their neighbours had been promised a cinema and community facility on that land, this set me to looking on a map and sure enough the map showed all that area to be Wyken Green. Thus was the Wyken Green Club formed! No allies were to be found in our parents, the value of property going up as the facility of most use to the kids, wild waste land with no supervision, was cut down. There were several gangs who took exception to the destruction of the open range but we were the only club with written rules, subs and the pledge, no pasaran. This last a guarantee of failure, we knew we would lose in the end but were determined to carry on a guerrilla operation for as long as we were able and to engage the enemy as others have said, by all means possible.

The other gangs would wait for the brick-layers to finish their work and go and push as many of the newly erected walls over as possible, nice enough tactically and action that slowed down the dirty work considerably, the police were often called and a watchman employed to hang around and watch the newly erected brickwork. The efforts of the gangs were called 'mindless vandalism' by the mindless who could not, or perhaps, would not see what the younger element had to lose. The club's efforts were, generally much more subtle or perhaps cunning and consequently more effective though positively dangerous at times. Dad commented that the club would be better called, 'The Winson Green Club, the way you lot carry on, because that's where you'll end up', Winson Green being a prison in Birmingham.

One of my suggestions was the misaligning of the trenches for the footings, achieved by moving the pegs put in for the next day's digging, this I had to supervise as the tendency was for others to move the things in such a way that it would be obvious that they had been moved. A couple of inches short, long or to one side was much better, and caused many delays and arguments. One of the major undertakings was intelligence, we had to know when the watchman went to the pub as this made life easier. So a watch would be kept until his predictable time-table was known.

A strategically placed hole in the pipe carrying the water to the site could be quite casually achieved even under general scrutiny, I shan't reveal how, and could bleed for hours before anyone was any the wiser whereas an axe through the thing would be noticed straight away and I will say now that when the axing happened it was nothing to do with me or W. G. C. Axing was too crude and almost certain to lead to the unpleasant and deleterious consequences of being caught.

Chapter 42

Careful breaking of things was another matter, if everything seemed good and usable until it came round to deploying it, more time would be lost, a weakened wooden component, a slightly cracked pipe, a window fastener bent out of true, these were W. G. C. trademarks.

'Attacks' on the person of the watchman was our other defensive tactic, someone amongst us owned a replica flintlock pistol and a penny banger would be shoved down the barrel when the poor old devil came into sight, watching away trying to catch us red-handed, the banger would be lit and the handgun carefully aimed, this would get the watchman dodging and throwing up his arms to protect his face, the banger would bang and he would seek cover yelling....well it was difficult to say what, but yelling, when we would melt away. Needless to say nothing shot toward him, but sparks and smoke made it seem a very realistic threat. That was the gun and no real threat, but the bazooka was, this weapon was a cardboard tube which had formerly contained a poster, sent appropriately through the post, one end was securely blocked and the other open, a sky rocket would be lit, dropped into the tube and fired in the general direction of the watchman, this frightened all concerned but he was never hit on the few occasions it was used but the gun terror enhanced his uncertainty. Children, please don't try this at home!

Tragedy came to W. G. C. in the form of a weapon developed by me with assistance from Al. This was a firebomb constructed from two tins one slightly smaller than the other so that it fitted into the larger tin which was equipped with a length of wire formed into a handle at one end the other tightly tied around the tin, on hitting the ground the small tin broke free and the contents of both tins scattered. The smaller tin had several lines of holes punched round from top to bottom, the mixture was then placed in the larger tin and lit, the smaller tin was then jammed on and the two tins whirled around the head to gain momentum and then let fly at the target, the tins separated and the contents were scattered where they burned for a few minutes, a great many trials were carried out and the tins always separated despite my fear that they would land in such a way that they remain attached. The mixture we used really proved a triumph, the tragedy was that we could not use the weapon as we wished, on the stock of wood and window frames inside a wire compound, as the conditions had changed, everyone else had given up and we were too well known to escape what would have been a very serious offence.

Gerry Northern lived as though he were a naturalised alien; he ate only ham or chips and if you were at his place his mother would ask what you want for your tea Gerry, ham or chips. One birthday he invited several of us to his party, and apart from the usual party treats, one could have ham or chips, most of us had neither. At the party we had the benefit of a novel sound system, an old wind-up gramophone, painted a violent sky blue in homage to the football club. These gramophones, already cluttering many an attic or garden shed and by now possibly sought after by collectors of early twentieth century electrical bygones, used metal needles to run in the grooves of the records and these had to be replaced frequently, the needle fitting into a lump of an electrical doo-dad fixed to a movable arm so that the needle could be placed by hand into the grooves. So Gerry turns the handle to wind the thing up places the needle in the groove while scratching the record by means of the spasms generated by his condition and away we go, before the record ends the music begins to slow and the voices to slur, Gerry furiously winds the handle again, all of us agog at such an antique way of providing entertainment, when the lump at the end of the arm complete with needle suddenly falls onto the record and is flung off by the spinning turntable to land on the floor needle first and stick there quivering. Gerry shouts that it's come off again and his mother comes in plucks the assemblage from the lino jams it back onto the arm and restarts the record which is now so scratched by all that it has gone through that it isn't worth listening to. The only guests Gerry had were W.G.C. members, in retrospect another indication of his isolation.

We never got to return to a refurbished Cleaver Ward at Gulson, because now the boy's side ward was on the ground floor, at the end of Fennell Ward in the place where the balcony had been on both Sage and Cleaver.

On Fennell the boy's ward was at the end of the men's through double doors where, on other wards, the balcony would be. On one side the bathroom on the other a small room full of trolleys, equipment, bandages etc. with a door to the outside.

Sister Sue Lyons transferred to Fennell along with other members of staff from Cleaver including the nurse who had an unfortunate crush on me when Cleaver temporarily moved to Whitley and two auxiliary nurses, Alma an Afro-Caribbean and Mrs Hopper, auxiliary nurses nowadays would be called nursing assistants no doubt.

I had during my time on Fennell great difficulty around what I saw as the practicalities and ethics of sex, my overwhelming need fought with my strong aversion to using and being used, I had always been a romantic and a 'brief encounter' would have been destructive to my sense of self at the time although something I would have enjoyed, besides didn't I love Denise and the thought of being unfaithful or rather disloyal to my idealised and cherished future mate was awful to contemplate, even though she had by that time told me that we had no future, my haemophilia ruling out life together but that I could ask anything else except permanence, still I had hope.

Though tempted to settle for the 'anything' I knew that would not be enough. The tremendous, unsettling obsession with sex awoke a dreadful fear that I would be so overcome by happiness and pleasure that I'd forget all ethical considerations to prolong the relationship and a worse fear that if, or rather when, she finally brought it to an end I would not be able to cope without continuing daily access........

I asked Mum to bring Denise to see me and one visiting time there she was, the visit wasn't without difficulty and I wished she could have come on her own, I couldn't say so, Mum would have been upset and Denise's parents would not have let it happen anyway.

She had asserted that we hadn't a future together and this tainted the pleasure I felt in her company and kept me in a dual state of wanting and not wanting to be even more attached to a loved person who would one day leave me. Despite this it was wonderfully soothing to know there was still a connection.

Had she been on her own I could have spoken freely, or as freely as I could let myself but it didn't happen and she never visited again.

A boy from school's mother, who visited each evening wearing a big fur coat, had a withered arm, perhaps from a stroke or maybe an accident and she gave off a peculiar smell. I commented on this to Mum, 'Don't be like that, it's a shame with that bad arm she can't look after herself.' I thought this unlikely but a typical piece of reasoning by Mum, on the other hand perhaps something about the female anatomy and its upkeep required both hands. As I write this now a big grin is on my face recalling how I finally grasped, a number of years later, that this lady had been misrepresented, the weird animal stink emanated from the fur coat, a laughter provoking revelation on getting too close to a fur stole about the shoulders of a 'lady' of seedy elegance!

Life with my parents often threw up laughter causing situations, mishearing and misuse of words. At the time of the 'fur coat and no knickers' accusation, Mum made another blunder by not listening to what I said, this was next day when I reported the curious and amusing phrase that another boy came out with concerning the fur furnished one. 'I don't like his mummy, she keeps chewing something.' This had made me smile and I assumed Mum would likewise think it funny, but a sad, chastened expression appeared on her face and she muttered 'It's only a bit of gum.' and took from her mouth a minute piece of chewing gum, wrapped it in paper and slipped it into her handbag. As I realised she thought the 'mummy' involved was her I was overcome by half-suppressed laughter and had to hide my face in the pillow. For the rest of the visit and for many days after, the image of her troubled face had me laughing again.

The few visits to Fennell were the last times I spent in hospital on children's or boys wards and were not without incident.

Most of the time the only other boy on the ward and I read, reading helps you move out of hospital to wherever the book is taking you, and time passed in this way brings you closer to discharge. There were only the two of us at first but one day a younger boy was admitted to the bed opposite mine, we talked with him for a while exchanging names and talking about the part of the city each lived. He was able to get up and about and was very active for someone admitted to a hospital ward.

When my companion and I decided to read the younger boy was not pleased and kept trying to distract us into talking, when that failed he took it as great fun to disturb the reading by suddenly running to the foot of our beds in turn and jumping onto the cross bar at the bottom, disrupting the flow of the reading with the sudden shock of being dragged back to the reality of the ward. Asked to stop, he just grinned, waited for us to get back to reading and started again. Then he was told to stop in no uncertain terms and we both promised him a shock if he tried it again.

Chapter 43

Being an old hand at the hospital lark I knotted the end of my towel and my neighbour did the same, equipped to make it more difficult for the aggressor next time. I, at least, hoped he'd take the hint and let me get back to my book. The threat proved no deterrent and the silly boy tried again, this time to be whacked by knotted towels, this made it even more fun for him unfortunately and it became a game, with him running in and dodging the swipes more often than not, eventually he tired and became easier to hit, so the game came to an end, and we went back to reading.

Towards the end of visiting time the kid started crying, as many did at the first visiting time when they knew that their visitors were about to leave. Suddenly Sister was sent for and his parents accused us of bullying him. Asked if we had hit him with knotted towels I said yes but only when he had jumped onto the end of the bed when we were reading and after he'd been asked not to do it. That's bullying the rather thick father said. In retrospect I should not have replied as I did, that all he had to do is leave us alone. This was interpreted as a threat and what I should have said was all he has to do is stop jumping on the end of the bed in order to annoy and provoke. If you've read this far you will know I have many things to be ashamed of, this is not one of them. I could have spent my time entertaining this boy, but I had my own way of coping and his way was up to him to find, not for his fellow patients to provide. He was transferred to Sage next day.

When settled down for the night, but not yet asleep we would often hear stealthy movements in the trolley room and often one of the night-nurses would go in there. There was a door to the outside and this opened outwards and should have been locked and only opened in an emergency, but we realised that someone was entering and keeping an assignation with this nurse. This was too good an opportunity to miss, and although we were confined to bed and both sets of legs were weak, we went into the room found a long bandage, tied it to several trolleys and to the outer door's handle, got back into bed and waited. A beautiful plan that worked so well, as the nurse shut the door behind her, it being all in darkness she failed to see the bandaging, the outer door was jerked open, a speedy tryst obviously being necessary, and a train of trolleys crashed and smashed about with falling kidney dishes and various other objects hitting the floor and adding to the cacophony. Our nurse yelped, 'for the love of God', a few further words were whispered, the door shut again, and a frantic tidying up began. We never heard a word about it and the clandestine visits ceased. Naughty boys no doubt, but the door should not have been left open, and that would be the reason we were never challenged about our trick.

Although confined to bed I was allowed to visit the w c in a wheelchair, after a nurse came to administer a suppository and I refused because all that was necessary to get a yes to the daily interrogation, 'Have you had your bowels open', was to let me position myself on the porcelain, 'You must have it, Doctor Butler ordered it,' Butler was the doctor whose duty was to hang around the ward, he was Irish so the nurses loved him, my reply was brutal but typical, 'Give it to him then'. Once again I was designated, 'a bold boy'. My suggestion as to Butler and the suppository may or may not have been taken up but mercy prevailed and my wheelchair suggestion was accepted and put in place immediately, very sensible and a big relief as I detested bed-pans ever since the shock of being made to use the things in public at Paybody.

Now we reach one of the places in this biography where matters become hard to believe, so I will present the facts as I know them and any reader who challenges them in any way is, of course, free to do so. I had a reputation as a fortune-teller and at that time on two separate occasions nurses came to me in a worried state for me to reveal what fate held. 'You read the cards, please help me'. On both occasions I somehow said the right words and both went away smiling. These skills, if such they were, came naturally to me not through my extensive reading or tuition.

I had an enemy on the ward, a staff nurse, determined to blame me for many things, none of which I had actually done. I still loved to make things in Plasticene, and sometimes these models were used by me to visualise things I wanted to happen. The model I made concerning my enemy grew as it went along, there was nothing planned or even an idea of what the final scene would show. I knew nothing of witchcraft or voodoo, but the first element was a model of the staff-nurse in her blue uniform white pinafore and white starched cap. Then I constructed a gallows, hung her from it and placed two dogs under her looking up and waiting for blood. Finally I stuck a pin through the left arm, and then placed the whole scene on my locker. Matron, on her daily visit, looked at it, smiled and said what a good model. The staff-nurse had a day off and didn't see it, but all the other nurses did, and several times I was called bold boy!

Staff-nurse, it transpired, had been involved in an accident but came back to work after one more day. She came into the room, her left arm in a sling, stood by my bed and snarled, 'You devil'. She gave no further trouble, a coincidence, yes? If no, then the tremendous luck I've had so many times requires no explanation.

The last discharge from Fennell was the last time I left Gulson Road Hospital and the last time I saw Sister Sue Lyons who's care of me and generally efficient running of the ward were exemplary. Now the hospital that played such a big part in my life has been demolished together with the nurse's home, the porter's lodge and all the ancillary buildings. The hospital that saved my life and witnessed the birth of my niece and the deaths of my infant siblings, the hospital where I was shown, almost invariably, love, compassion and care is gone.

As substantial, as permanent, as it seemed in my childhood, my second home, as Mum called it, has been completely erased, my beloved balconies gone for scrap, even the length of very old, broad sandstone wall, which as a boy I thought must be a remaining part of the city wall, with an appropriate growth of wallflowers, gone as if it never existed. Most of the people too, regretted but no longer here to be thanked as I wish I had, so long ago. So many names lost, so much kindness to remember, I thank them now.

Dad had promised to buy me a shed, this promise being made some years earlier he eventually repented or his tardiness and purchased, erected, painted, and fixed metal splash guards to keep the rain off the lowest three tongue and groove planks of the walls, later he added an opening window in the side as the interior got so hot, on the sunnier days. The shed was furnished with bookshelves, a small table, an old metal bed-settee for sitting, an old dining chair so that I could sit in front of the window and write, a paraffin heater and later a paraffin stove on which to heat up soup etc. and a dartboard. Various displays and collections such as fossils and a deconstructed 303 rifle shell mounted on a card with all parts labelled, this being one of the several I dug up on The Dump, also the fruits of my short-lived butterfly collection. The wall was scrawled with quotations from Shakespeare, Lewis Carroll, Omar Khayyam and the romantic poets, plus anything else that appealed to me. This was now our headquarters and on occasion I converted the settee to a bed and slept down there on hot summer nights.

Dad's other promise, which was never kept, or should I say disastrously made and atrociously never kept was one he had repeatedly made to me since I was not long out of Corley: You'll never have to search for a job, you'll come to Coventry Sheet Metal and take over the office, that's one of the reasons I started the business in the first place. As I had never seen why anyone should bother to employ me when bleeds would always intervene to prevent me attending work, just as they had school, this took a weight from my very young shoulders, an antidote to the fear of the future that had dogged me ever since I'd been given the book When I Grow Up and seen how many jobs would be impossible for me, and how uninviting to me those that were possible. It gave me a warm feeling to know that Dad understood and was doing his best to help. I was to be disillusioned.

Al and Derek; we had a signal, a whistle that would tell if both were out in our respective back gardens, if yes we would meet out in the entry and decide what to do with whatever time we had, some of the things were plain dangerous and some fun.

The compost experiment was an idea of pure genius as we knew very little about anaerobic composting as opposed to aerobic, we had the notion to make holes in a baby-milk-tin, fill the thing with green leafy material and grass, cramming it in, and then to bury it with a three-inch covering of earth. After a month we dug it up again and were astonished to see how far the leaves and grass had rotted, the material now taking up only a fifth of the space and having the texture and smell of well-rotted compost. This experiment was tried again but this time we dug it up after only two weeks and found it well on its way to becoming compost. We took it down to only one week and while this was not enough time to call the material anything close to compost it was, even after so short a time, beginning to break down quite well. We should have taken things further, moving the burial site, burying deeper or shallower, but sadly this did not happen.

We used to watch Percy Thrower's Gardening Club every week and discuss. We both started gardening inspired by Percy and I created a small rock garden with a pond made from an old sink, while Al made a bed of perennials. The other T V program we watched each week was Play for Today and we would drool over the acting and more especially the use of language, I recall those early Dennis Potter plays, Stand Up Nigel Burton and Vote, Vote, Vote for Nigel Burton, a couple of theatre of the absurd things whose names I forget, and a play called Drums Along The Avon, racialism and echoes of slavery. How could I get close to forgetting the natural history documentaries? David Attenborough's various Zoo Quests, Armand and Michaela Denis and many others.

Al and his brother Roy had made a soap-box trolley and Al took it up onto The Dump and rode it down the slope, it looked such fun, but when he pulled it back up and asked if I wanted a turn I said no. I didn't trust the track which sloped two ways, down and slightly across and I could see that the possibility of overturning was just on the side of sixty-forty not my kind of odds. Al took off down the slope a second time and while it is true to say that the trolley didn't overturn, what it did was just as bad, it tipped to one side enough to bring Al's backside into contact with the track and kept on sliding down to the bottom. The track was not smooth and had stones and bits of brick sticking out of it, Al's jeans were ripped and he was in considerable pain, though the skin wasn't broken, and he disentangled himself and limped about rubbing his thigh and backside. The cart was never brought out again.

Bombs were a big part of our manufacture, and we progressed to guns as well. Penny bangers were good in those days and contained quite a lot of black-powder, incidentally we found out that the tuppenny bangers did not have twice as much and a bit more as we had hoped but contained the same amount but the tube was twice as thick. Our own bombs were improved by this knowledge as wrapping our containers round and round with sticky tape or encasing them with papier mache and allowing it to dry gave more explosive power for our powder expenditure. The bombs were a great success as no-one was injured but people were astonished to hear such loud explosions with so little damage and we learned a lot from the various mixes we used with the base of black-powder. We discovered that the addition of sugar produced an explosion a little less violent than we would have wished but a massive amount of black smoke, we set one off at the bottom of my garden just as Mum came out of the back-door I shouted to her to wait there a moment, the thing blew and an enormous mushroom cloud of smoke rose over the garden. Mum told anyone who would listen that I'd made a thing like a nuclear bomb. Dad told me to be careful.

We also took delight in making sodium flares with sodium chlorate weed killer and sugar; we were never tempted to use this mixture in our bombs because of its inherent instability.

Chapter 44

We would make a pile of the mixture at night and ignite it by throwing on a match when it would burn with high intensity light, enough to make it like day in the immediate area and we experimented with the shape of the pile of material to get the longest burn without losing the intensity.

Our first attempt at a gun was nearly our last and potentially a disaster for Al. I found a piece of two-by-two timber and cut a deep groove with one end open, and placed in it a piece of steel tube in which we made a small touch hole. The tube was pushed tight up to the end of the groove with the touch hole on the upper surface and held in place by strips of tin, the first firing went well, but the next blew back as Al knelt to light the priming powder and a chunk of the wood smacked him on the forehead and his face was blackened. Fortunately no real damage was done but the gun project was put on hold until we could acquire a better gun barrel. A boy who lived a couple of doors away from my Gran took to coming round and one day after looking at my collection of rounds of ammunition he brought me a present of a small anti-aircraft shell, at least that's what he'd been told it was but I quickly discovered that it was a model and had been turned on a lathe from a piece of bronze, was hollow and had a plug at the base which could be removed.

Gun mark two, we unscrewed the plug and discarded it, made a hole for the priming powder at the sharp end, fitted the thing into another prepared piece of two-by-two, putting in a domed tap washer between the end of the barrel and the closed end of the carriage to take up some of the recoil and again bound up the whole thing with strips of metal, more of them and a couple of thou thicker, the closed end of the tube preventing an accident similar to the one that led to the demise of mark one. This time the thing worked perfectly, when muzzle loaded with black powder, wadding and a ball-bearing, or a couple of dozen air gun pellets. After each firing, now initiated by a fuse made of solid fuel igniter used for rocket powered models aircraft we carefully cleaned and realigned the gun. We stuffed a tin with leaves and sand mixed together and fired our pellets, at it, the tin was knocked backwards and several of the pellets had gone right through and come out the other side. When we used the ball-bearing we fired it at a sheet of thick plywood, the ball went straight through and hit Gerald Houghton's bike which had been left against the fence about fifteen feet away, the bike went flying and we never found the ball-bearing but on examination the bike frame had a perfectly round dent which penetrated to a depth half the size of the missile. This experiment had drawn a crowd which we were careful not to let happen again as one of the idiots suddenly stood in front after we had lit the fuse, I barked at him to get out of the way, waving him to the side and he hesitated only to comply at the last moment. He could have lost a leg as the ball would have been at knee height by the time it got to where he was standing. Instead, Gerald's bike bore the scar. We used sand to elevate the gun and this worked very well, also the barrel would move forward a little on firing as the domed washer took the force, deformed, sprang back and pushed the barrel forward.

Mum's sister, christened Dora but always called Flo had always been a favourite of mine and yearly, in late Spring, paid us a visit, she lived in Hinckley which meant a bus ride to Coventry and the another bus to Wyken where we lived and for Aunt Flo this had to be on a sunny pleasant day. We would receive a letter in which she would say she was coming to see us soon as there was a nice day. There would be several 'nice' days and then one morning I would awake knowing that today Aunt Flo was coming and tell Mum, she'd tell me that just because it was a nice day it didn't mean Aunt Flo would come. I knew she was coming and was there to open the door to her when she arrived. Mum would tell of her surprise at my being right and Aunt Flo would laugh, a thing she did regularly. As a child I would start jumping around and she would always say: Don't get excited lad, don't get excited. Mind the Axminster! Often she brought me a little toy, once a flimsy plastic racing car with a hole on top through which protruded a balloon, the end of the balloon emerged from the rear of the car after it passed through an assemblage holding a perforated disc. The balloon could be inflated, pinched at the point where it left the body of the car, placed on the floor, the balloon released and the whole thing would shoot down the room jet powered by air while the disc spun round and made a piercing zooming sound, an ingenious toy, and the spinning disc assembly would give me hours of non-innocent fun once the toy racing car and balloon had gone the way of all flimsy toys.

My parents had always used me as an excuse when asked if they had been on holiday, no holiday because Derek always has a bleed. This was not strictly true and the only thing my haemophilia had cocked-up was a day out at Skegness, just when I didn't need it as I'd invited Denise to go with us and was looking forward to a trip on the funfair's Tunnel of Love, Sapristi, foiled again! The other curious thing was that as we had to get up very early to make this trip worthwhile, Dad had put in enough petrol to get us well into the journey and someone had entered the garage and siphoned off the petrol, a thing that had never been known before. They must have known says Dad and everyone who knew about our trip came under suspicion. That, as far as I know, was the only time a bleed had disrupted Mum and Dad's plans.

Mum's niece Frances had married a Lincolnshire man, Ken, they had one daughter and though I must have met them before, my first memory of them all is when I first came home from Corley. I remember visiting the old farm cottage they lived in at the time, and marvelling at the pump in the kitchen which emptied into the stone sink, and being delighted to meet Carol. Ken was a farm worker with laughter in his soul, his eyes crinkled up and his cheeks reddened as he found yet another thing hilarious he was altogether a good friend and a conscientious man. Frances was not severe exactly and could be very pleasant, but had a nervous side to her character which often seemed to put her on the edge of temper and as Ken and Carol both bit their nails her irritation would be manifested by a sudden, loud and grating, 'Ken!' or 'Carol!', startling everyone in the room. Even the budgie in his cage would be yelled at, in the same manner, every time he attempted to preen, the explanation given being that he was 'feather-picking', I dare say the poor bird achieved his feather maintenance when not under scrutiny and suspect that Frances' intolerance was more to do with her nerves. She was always very pleasant to me for which I remain grateful especially as I must have been annoying too, at times. Carol delighted me and I wanted to get to know her much better. Carol's paternal grandparents lived in Orby Lincolnshire, and a few times we holidayed with them, my memory tells me that Carol would spend most of the school summer holidays with them.

The house was fascinating to me as it had no mains utilities and was like a glimpse of the past, with oil lamps for light and little Kelly lamps to place on the bedside cabinet while one undressed and got into bed.

I think the water came via a pump in the kitchen, but don't remember ever seeing it or going into the kitchen, the large pantry I looked into once and there were hooks for hams, or so I was told, cooking was often done on the large range in the living-room cum kitchen and water for tea was always boiled there, in the kitchen was the only concession to modernity, a bottled-gas cooker. I now believe that the room referred to as the kitchen was in fact a scullery in the past and that the room with the range was a farmhouse style kitchen. There wasn't a water closet but an outside privy with a holed plank and a bucket underneath, this was the ancient arrangement but of course it was new to me, so I tried not to use it, preferring to wait until we were out in Skegness to find a w c. There was a pig-sty in the garden, but never a pig, and a long vegetable garden and orchard. Of the several rooms upstairs one was used to store apples and maybe pears, but I remember the apples each one half-wrapped in newspaper and covering the surface of a trestle table, the sash window always slightly open to keep the room cool and permit the circulation of air.

What I liked most was crossing over a little bridge to get onto the property leaving modernity and entering the past each time we arrived.

We would drive into Skegness most days and walk across the less than blazing desert to the sea, which had receded so far that for most of the walk dry sand impeded me and soon got into whatever footwear I had on, it seemed like miles and I soon lost interest in the Skegness sea experience. The fun fair owned by Billy Butlin was another story.

Chapter 45

The ghost train, which was never so much frightening as irritating when scratchy bits of string hit you in the face, what this was thought to simulate Butlin himself would be hard-pressed to say. It was dark, and had a weird smell to it but I liked to ride it with Carol. My other favourite was the Tunnel of Love although its official title was something like Water Caves, you entered little two-seater boats and the artificial flow of the water took you into the mouth of a simulated cave for a few minutes ride through the dark, the smell was different to the Ghost Train but just as weird. This ride too was better when accompanied by Carol. The rest of the fun fair was the usual stuff, being exhorted to waste money by tossing rings or throwing at coconuts but the worst thing was the so-called Zoo that I visited often in order to be appalled, which is of course as necessary to any primate's experience as warmth, sustenance and shelter.

The Zoo did not smell weird, it stank. It was a large room with glass-fronted cages wherein mangy, retired old lions served out their time, lying down looking not at all regal but slightly moth eaten, the oldest specimen having only half a tail. I also recall a non-moving porcupine, but the creatures I spent most time looking at were an ever expanding colony of rhesus monkeys, over the three or so years I visited them they spread to three of the glass fronted cages, but were still over-crowded and I couldn't watch them for long, monkey society seemed to be reduced to chaos with females pulling their babies off the teat and casually dropping them to the floor where they would sit crying out for their mothers while getting knocked over and trampled by the mob charging around after the lucky one who had found a piece of fruit in the sawdust covering the base of the cage. Always one, or perhaps two, monkeys would be sitting against the wall either trying to sleep, or die. The females were given no rest and were mated with over and over again, and in retrospect I feel the colony was diseased, as strips of skin hung down from the backsides of many of them. I hated the Zoo but was at the same time fascinated by it and always paid it a visit hoping to see an improvement in the animal's conditions. No-one seemed to agree that the idea of keeping these wretched animals indoors without natural light or anything to stimulate them was cruel. Many years later I visited again but the whole fun fair had been pulled down.

Sex and violence or rather sex, and later violence was on offer in the building next to the fun fair entrance, this was one-story and made of concrete, windowless with gaudy semi-nude pictures of harem girls painted on the walls and had the title Arabian Nights. People under twenty-one were not allowed in and parents were reluctant to answer questions about what went on inside. Mostly they'd evade an answer by saying you'll have to wait until you're twenty-one. This was, I suppose, tableaux where nude women were allowed to pose as long as they did not move, a curious compromise that lasted some years in this country. Then all this was swept away, the nudes white-washed and a new thrill for the masses took over, this time it was all about Japanese atrocities during wartime and the outside illustrations had lots of bamboo, samurai swords, bloody prisoners and yelling guards. The twenty-one restriction stood but this time the people on the outside didn't hurry the kids past as quickly as they had when a glimpse of nipple through lacy clothing might have upset them and corrupted their poor defenceless children.

The other attraction, one I actually liked was called the Waterways, this was a system of canals that wound through municipally planted gardens, some on little islands, and eventually brought you back to the start. The little power boats didn't go very fast but you had to take control and guide them through the maze of canals. This was a good ride unlike so many others, being outside where at least the smells were identifiable, and one could savour these or not as one chose and enjoy the sound of less fortunate juniors begging their parents for a go.

The other fascinating thing was that a great many crabs lived in the waters of the canals and were easily caught. The technique learned from watching others required three essentials, string long enough to reach the bottom of the canal, a stone capable of being tied to the string and a shrimp, less essential but very useful were a bucket of the bucket and spade variety. The stone had to be knobbly, a regular pebble would slip out from the string, people were always chucking half eaten packets of shrimp down and so bait was readily available. The stone was tied to the string with the shrimp roughly three inches above, the assemblage was then lowered into the water until the stone hit bottom, the string kept taught and after a short while a grab by a crab, the equivalent of a fisherman's bite, would be made and when you felt it tugging you slowly and gently pulled the string and out of the depths appeared the crab gamely hanging on to its catch, a steady calm pull got the crab just under the surface, if you let it break the surface at that point it would let go and you had to start again. This time you got it to the same point just under the surface.... and then......snatched and with luck the crab held on too long and landed on the bank, his job then was to scuttle back into the water while we tried to stop him and if we succeeded have a good look before allowing him to sidle back and dive in. This is where a bucket could be useful as it was possible to capture him, examine at leisure before releasing back to his home environment.

Gibralter point I remember with affection for its sand dunes, wild birds and dangerous looking seas, not that the waves would have interested a surfer particularly, but that they seemed to lack a certain predictability reaching shore from two directions in a boiling chaos in tune with the wildness of the place. The briskness of the wind once out of the protection of the dunes was an irresistible force, the gulls arrowing with it then turning to battle, rising up and up.

We also had our picnic there in the dunes, and I didn't want to leave partly because of the golf course where, just a couple of weeks prior, a man walking by had been struck by a golf ball and killed, or at least that's what Ken said as we ate our picnic. I had noticed a curious thing many times previously, if any ball was struck, with foot or bat or thrown with force it would immediately take a line towards me so until we were clear of the wretched golf course I stood in danger.

One holiday at Orby we had bed and breakfast in a nearby farmhouse. Most of my breakfasts at the farmhouse were uneventful and all the more enjoyable for it as eating is what breakfast is for, but one morning was interrupted by a strange yet strangely normal display of the way my parents interacted. Dad suddenly complained there was something wrong with his egg, all three had soft-boiled eggs; Mum took a look and told him it was addled and that it sometimes happened if the hens lay away, I'll get Mrs Glover to bring you another one. Snaps Dad, 'No, don't.' and with shaking hand thrusts it at Mum 'Here you eat it'! 'Don't be so daft, I'm not eating an addled egg for you.' and before he could stop her she rings the bell we've been given, Mrs Glover comes, takes away the offending egg coming back in a few minutes with another, Dad looks as though he wishes he could squash himself down into total insignificance, Mum says thank you, and once the door is closed shakes her head and tells him, and me what a funny man he is.

Mum would often arrive home with crusty rolls and home cured ham or pork also home-cooked. So many times our eating of these was relatively normal apart from Dad's usual eye movements, suspicious I suppose that Mum or I were watching to see how the self-conscious man of the house would manage a crusty roll.

But one gloriously silly day the roll as he bit into it bit back and trapped his lip and he couldn't get it loose. It clung on and pinched him. It could have been wrenched off but would certainly have cut his lip. He told us it was stuck, Mum told him what a funny man he was, and offered no assistance. He turned to me saying 'Derek!' and I stood and told him to sit still while I found the right place to squeeze the roll. It had mercy and released its grip, never get these rolls again he told Mum, 'Well' she said 'I've never heard of anyone getting bitten by a roll before'. Several weeks went by with no further incident until.......that's right it happened again, this time the operation to remove the beast was a little more tricky as a tiny bit of his tongue was involved, but by careful manipulation I triumphed once more. 'I told you not to get these bloody things again!' Then he gave a sheepish smile and said 'I don't know! I'm the picture of bad luck'.

If you think I'm very negative about my father, think again, the notice I took of his utterances and actions shows how much I loved the man and how hard I tried to understand him. To me, when young, he seemed to be the epitome of someone capable of seeing a task through to the end, and of a deep integrity, only later I apprehended him as highly self-conscious, partly my own nature but much watered down.

Holidays were enlivened because Al joined us, I'm not sure how many of these there were but I do remember two. The first of these was at Weymouth and was very eventful, I say this was the first but I may be running two holidays together, Mum, Dad Al and I shared a very small caravan at Litlesea Caravan Park, the little sea in the name being the Fleet, a brackish linear lake trapped between the Chesil Beach and the land, it stank as I remember probably from sewage outfall but the view across to Chesil Beach made up for it. The site had a complex with a shop, and entertainment building, showers and toilet facilities.

The caravan we hired had the name It'll Do Us on the side and the previous year had been hired by Ron and Mary and their daughter Frances, Mary was my Dad's cousin but since I was a kid I'd been encouraged to think of them as my aunt and uncle and Frances as my cousin. This year they had a larger van and had brought Frances's friend with them, I don't remember her name but she was given the nickname Weather-Cock, I have absolutely no idea why. At the time I was a butterfly collector and Al assisted me in chasing after various fritillaries with absolutely no result, these insects were very fast flying and may well have all been the same, as we never got close to them it remains an open question. On a trip to Lulworth Cove I did catch a Lulworth Skipper but very soon after that I gave collecting up as it was not a scientific investigation and butterflies were beginning to suffer because of changes in farming and other pressures and I did not want to add to their decline even in a small way.

On this holiday we drank illegally bought vodka and chased around after female members of our own species, not just butterflies, without a great deal of success but diligently. There were two girls in particular who caught our fancy; we never even got to find out their actual names. We knew them as Pixie and Beebee.

Chapter 46

Pixie because she had that impish kind of face that I liked with short blonde hair, and Beebee because she had big breasts, our problem was that we both preferred Pixie and as the two appeared always together we were torn and with the arrogance of youth imagined they would be torn too.........

I still longed for Denise but when she came over to see me when several of my mates were there I felt under pressure, one of them said fuck, and I immediately tried to apologise but she said, it's alright that's what I wanted to talk to Derek about, cleverly said because they shut up completely. The outcome was not so wonderful because now I felt embarrassed that she had been so open in front of them, I was in a very bad way at the time, confused and unsure but by then everything seemed to torture me and I could never forget her assertion that my haemophilia would one day part us. My life had involved me in too many decisions at too young an age, and haemophilia had played a big part in that as other people didn't seem to understand my difficulties and fear of being stranded somewhere with a bleed and reliant on people who hadn't a clue how to treat the situation. I might well be dragged into a hospital, perhaps of the cottage variety where nothing would be done until I could persuade the staff to contact Parry-Williams. That would have been a real challenge back then. Al's grandparents offered to let me stay for part of the summer holidays with Al in Wales and the idea was tempting, I would have enjoyed the change, but I had to say no, and was astonished that anyone, most especially my parents, couldn't see the potential for disaster.

One other holiday with my parents and Al deserves a mention, Dad bought a large frame tent as did Ron and Mary, and we camped at a splendidly rural site near Swanage, three tents because Uncle Sam came with us and had a small tent of his own. The two girls, Frances and Weather-Cock, used to like to go into his tent and giggle at each other, one sunny afternoon another chuckling voice joined in their giggles and Al and I walking past exchanged glances, the door-flap opened and out popped Uncle Sam who said a shocking thing through a big grin, 'You want to get in there, they're all the same size lying down!' We said nothing and ignored his advice.

Back at school things were beginning to reach a climax, my mates and I were now all prefects and were required to be alert to the disruptive efforts of younger boys. One of our duties was to supervise the boy's toilets and washroom during break. We would go in, tame any roughhousing, chuck out smokers and generally speed up the visits made by shooing them out straight after hands had been washed. Once the kids knew prefects were present our job was done and we could be about our own business. Spike had been eating and sharing a bar of chocolate, the milk chocolate he always referred to as, cheesy chocolate, and there were two squares left. None of us wanting to help him dispose of it by the usual method, he asked, 'What shall we do with it?' never a good idea to ask such a question with Derek available for consultation. Melt it on the radiator I said, the idea was taken up and gradually developed by committee, into a devilish scheme.

We melted the chocolate in a bit of the silver-paper wrapper until gooey, then smeared it on the wall of the washroom, using a piece of scratchy school toilet paper which we then left stuck in the chocolaty mess, a little artistic competence was needed to get the authentic look a faeces smearing disturbee would achieve. After a little drying time, one of the upright law-abiding prefects fetches the caretaker; this gentleman was appalled to think anyone could do such a thing as smear and goes off to equip himself with rubber gloves, and cleaning materials. He retches as he cleans what is after all only chocolate, turning his head away and complaining about the stink and retching some more. 'The dirty little devils, if I catch 'em... Mr Bulstrode won't have this'! Mercifully the bell sounded and we trooped off to lessons.

At this time, the careers officer interviewed each of us who were getting to the end of our school days, and in my case tether, and the question was put to me in the form of a statement: You'll have been thinking about what you want to do when you leave school. No I replied, and in outraged tones, not giving me time to explain, he told me, I must! I then explained that my father was a company director and had promised me a job in the firm, running the office, and that's why I had not worried about what I was going to do. In fact Dad told me one of his reasons for starting up the business was, 'So that you'll never have to worry about finding a job'. The careers officer said he would look into it and a course was arranged in typing, Pitman's shorthand, simple book keeping and general office skills. At the same time Dad dropped his bombshell, not to my face, but through Mum, stating that I shouldn't have told them I was going to work at Red Lane. I started my course however and during it the final blow-up between him and his partners took place.

My father's demands, to my way of thinking had become more and more unreasonable, he wanted Uncle Bob to leave his job which was close to getting him his superannuation and get his hands dirty doing physical work at Red Lane. One night Uncle Bob crossed the road and came to talk, Dad was all controlled aggression and Bob turned to leave, at the door he looked back spread his arms, palms up and said to me,' I'll come to Red Lane as soon as I've got my superannuation, I can't say fairer than that, can I Derek'? Dad jumped up, wild eyed and stood like an animal at bay, 'You leave Derek out of this'! Bob shrugged and left the room and the house and as far as I know never entered again. Surely it was much too late to leave me out of it, after all it was Dad who'd brought me in? If Dad was king in his home then I was a pawn, that became clear to me, nothing was ever said to me directly about his failed intervention in my life, if such it was, I've since been informed that he made these promises to several others; back then I still hoped that he would somehow keep his promise to me not knowing at the time that one of his chief assets as a father and a man, overarching integrity, was a fantasy of mine.

Then he resigned his directorship, took cash payment including an agreed sum for the shares held in other companies and left the firm.

So there was I during my last months at school working away at a commercial course that had little to interest me apart from the phonetics of Pitman's shorthand and no paper qualification to be gained at the end of it. I had lessons in a room made available in top-school with all the little kids outside at break time taking great interest and looking in the window, until the novelty wore off, asking each other, is that Miss Stevens? Miss Stevens was the school secretary and I could only hope they meant Miss Castleton who had been brought into school specifically to teach me, but as I was the one typing I fear they meant me!

We got on well together and I don't remember ever being on the edge of losing my temper, we would work on the various aspects of my course, filing and simple book-keeping seemed, well, simple to the point of being boring and the typing was difficult because keeping my eye off the keyboard seemed too much like losing control. The shorthand fascinated me however and I only wanted to learn more. She would bring in an amusing magazine written in shorthand, and we would read that and practise using the few instructional bits, there would always be something to laugh about, but don't get the impression that hard work was ignored, far from it and you must remember that at that at the beginning I still hoped for a position in the family firm. Shorthand and office skills took up my mornings and after lunch my friends and me were allowed to study in the library, I don't know what Spike, Michael and Bruce were studying but none of the four spent much time on it, old habits die hard and Lewis Carroll, Shakespeare, Edward Lear and others would come into play, amid discussions of this that and a good part of the time the other, poetry, of a sort, would be made. These were the best times I spent at Baginton, which alas, I did not make a success of, but then the school failed to make a success of me

Shortly after this brief flirt with contentment I left school to carry on my commercial course at home, my parents being marvellously generous in letting us study in the living-room while they went out, where they went I have no idea but they usually returned just after Miss Castleton had left. This helpful gesture gave me the chance to finish my course and was well appreciated partially making up for the disappointment of not having a job to go to.

I have no recollection of my last day at school, no goodbyes or anything of that nature and believe that I must have been in hospital at the time or ill in bed, it would be very strange if I managed to forget such a transition after remembering so much. Two further incidents before I leave school behind in this episodic narrative.

Chapter 47

The draughts competition that I should have won, but refused to take part in was won by someone I could beat almost without trying, in retrospect this was a mistake on my part, and must go down as one of the drawbacks associated with not taking part in 'the life of the school'.

Just before Christmas one year a competition was organised, this involved a long list of general knowledge questions - something whispers five hundred, but that seems too many - the whole school took part and Al and I went to Kingsway Library for the answers we didn't immediately know. We both answered a great many of the questions but when it was time to hand in the paper I had a knee bleed and although Al offered to take my answers in for me, the fact that several questions remained unanswered I found hard to accept and turned down the offer. It may seem fictional but Al won. He came to tell me and told how he had revealed to the school that I should have won it as I'd many more answers than him. Did I regret refusing his offer? Yes, but I resented my haemophilia much more as it had prevented me making another trip to the library, a trip I had meticulously planned by writing down whereabouts I might find the illusive answers.

It was right and proper that Al should have won and a great boost for a wonderful mate and I hope my disappointment at not going for it allowed me to tell him so.

We shared an interest in gardening, and an enemy, the man my Dad called Sludge Guts who lived a few houses up the street. From my shed we could fire peas at the roof of his garage when we knew he was inside, he would come shambling out and look up in the trees suspecting, what? After a close inspection of nothing much he would go back into the garage, and after a minute or so we would redouble our efforts and out he would come again to gaze upwards, obviously perplexed as only 'a bear of very little brain' could be, a third volley sent him indoors and exhorting his wife to come and experience the phenomenon, this person had a loud and gobbling voice and we could hear her telling him not to be so silly and that she didn't have time for this. All highly satisfactory, but used this sparingly to keep his wondering interest.

So what had Sludge-Guts done to provoke our contempt? Dad always complained 'Sludge-Guts again.' when we drove round the entry to our garage and he and his car completely blocked the way as he washed or polished it. The man would have to back it into his garage to let us past, so slowly getting down to it that Dad would be muttering, to get a bloody move on. This is how

Sludge-Guts got his name, and his tooing and frowing, shambling and fumbling irritated me as well. His worst crime however, and the reason he became a target for torment was probably lost in the mists of time as far as he was concerned. He had once heard noises under his shed, which turned out to be hedgehogs, in a reasonably intelligent and compassionate person this would have been the end of it, but not Sludge-Guts, he had the useful creatures destroyed by pest control people, I despised him for this stupid overreaction and for the fact that he had set-up a horrible battery cage system for hens against the front of his shed. It was possible to see the hens from other gardens, their only protection a tarpaulin that was lowered over them at night, we kept chickens in an extensive run with a proper chicken-house for their comfort and protection, other people kept hens or ducks, but none of them felt the need to resort to cruel factory farming methods in their own gardens!

After a long bout of being off my legs because of bleeds I found it very difficult to walk more than a few paces indoors or out; muscle had been lost and my legs would start to tremble after only a short distance which meant never going out into the city or walking in the countryside and I knew action was needed, the unacceptable challenged. I decided on a program of walking to improve the muscles, my thinking being that legs were designed for walking so the best physiotherapy was to walk. Many years later I mentioned my theory to a physiotherapist and she reacted with horror, however the results were remarkable and I went on to improve my stamina and then my posture and the greatest help I received was from Al.

During the summer months of one year we took a walk together every day, a little further each time, and Al would wait patiently as I sat for a couple of minutes when the trembling of the muscles started. Time to pay respect to the neighbours who never once objected to my sitting on their front garden walls until I could carry on, gradually we managed to get further and further up the street by this incremental method, and slowly I began to need less rests along the way, Al stuck with me throughout the therapy and over the months my strength grew and pretty soon we increased the range to take in more streets and I found that eventually I could walk a long distance before the need to sit became unbearable, I also amusingly learned to mark sitting places far down the road and control my distress until I reached one, the fact that I went on from there to be able to walk all the way to my Gran's house without sitting is attributable to my own determination and the tenacity and true friendship of Al who never failed to accompany me through the initial stages.

In case you might be thinking that I only laughed at other people's misfortunes and mistakes, here's something that had me laughing uncontrollably at myself, so much so that Miss Castleton put her hand on my wrist and asked what the matter was, in such a sensitive manner that it made me laugh all the harder.

Wyken, and perhaps further afield, occupied the time and energy of a very dapper rag-and-bone man, always very smartly dressed, clean and tidy. My parents were having an extension built and I saw a besuited man poking about in the garden as I was taking down a passage in shorthand, I assumed it was the foreman of the building crew, counting bricks or whatever else such types do. A few seconds later a knock came on the back-door and on opening it this person said to me with a rising intonation, have you got any rag? Oh, God I thought why must we be constantly interrupted, I suppose Mum promised them rag to wipe their hands on, I rushed back indoors telling him I'd look, pulled open the drawer Mum used for cut up old clothes to be used as dusters and took out a couple of flannel sized pieces, strode back to the door and dropped them into his outstretched hand, he stood there with his hand out looking down at the measly largesse dispensed by a cruel and clownish young man, turned away, half-turned back and said, thank you. It wasn't until I got back to the typewriter that I realised my mistake and just couldn't stop laughing, the more concerned Miss Castleton became, the harder became the struggle to stop laughing at my idiotic bout of mistaken identity. Once I found it possible to explain she too found it hilarious.

There remains another incident from the time of my tuition, and this is one I still can't fathom, was she so carried away by our commercial studies that she forgot where she was, a provocation, or is there another explanation that I just haven't thought of. I was typing away and her hand suddenly went to the thigh nearest me and she hoisted her skirt right up so far that I could see stocking top, suspender, and a smooth, white portion of upper thigh, scratched idly with the other hand and after what was a short interval but seemed a long one lowered her skirt again, astonished I stopped typing and looked away when once more she asked me what was wrong. I couldn't tell her then but would give so much to experience the moment again when at least I could offer the courtesy of an explanation.

Miss Castleton gave me two objects, alas both of them lost when I left my first wife, but that whole episode will have to wait for my adult years biography, the first was a black leather pocket book with the original leaves of paper for notes and sections for stamps, cards etc. This had belonged to her father and although old seemed almost unused, the second object was more fun and she gave it to me with a laugh and the words, 'A little irreverent but never mind.' it was small prayer book covered in green leather and fastened with a tab and button, on opening it revealed itself as containing a pack of playing cards and had on the green leather front the words, Let Us Play, irreverent indeed and when you come to understand that she was secretary of her local church, quite unexpected. I almost forgot the most useful and badly needed thing she gave me, a large, old-fashioned bookcase, glass-fronted and well-made with the glass and wooden sections lifting up and back to reveal each shelf. The sad thing is I have no memory of how my books were kept before that, I assume they formed piles or lived on and in my bedside cabinet, the idea of providing accommodation for books was alien to my parents, who always seemed bemused and frightened by my catholic taste in, and love of books. That bookcase was one of the most significant gifts I ever received and was soon filled to overstretching.

She taught me well and although, apart from a brief interlude, I never used the skills in employment, not having a certificate to show prospective employers proved a real drawback as did the lack of A and O-levels, the phonetics enabled me to see the structure of the words I was reading and the confidence in typing has been a useful tool. I have no recollection of the day when my studies ended, but I know that I failed to keep in touch, a major failing of mine over the years in many situations, as I find it difficult to imagine why anyone would want to bother with me, half the time, and the rest feel too busy and productive to bother with them; a stultifying lack of self-confidence struggling with a surplus of energy and self-belief bordering on arrogance being the twin poles of my life. I remain grateful to Miss Castleton for actually teaching me something of value at secondary school.

The completion of my commercial course was like the leaving of Baginton Fields, a damp squib or more realistically a petering out.......

I learned very little, officially, at special school, a couple of 'dirty' songs, which I choose not to go into, a small number of facts, confirmation of my prejudices and beliefs and increased willingness to access an education should anyone be bothered to assist me.

So what did I learn overall from my journey through those often painful, often joyful years of gradual revelation? That it was possible, if my endurance could be stretched far enough, to outlast the bad times and the few toxic people who'd impinged. Most importantly, that I have many to thank for the care and love that got me through my first eighteen years. Years that left me emotionally damaged but with coping strategies fully developed, if aberrant, and an understanding of my physical capabilities and the limit to which I could safely push them. Thank you. Sorry.......

ND - #0242 - 080726 - C0 - 197/132/25 - PB - 9781780353197 - Gloss Lamination